LET FOOD BE YOUR MEDICINE

DR. STEVE'S GUIDE TO MANAGE YOUR HEALTH, AGING, DISEASE, AND WEIGHT GAIN

BY DR. STEVE KRINGOLD

EDITORIAL REVIEWS

In our modern society, the very essence of eating has transformed into a mere indulgence, prioritizing taste and convenience over nutrition. Dr. Kringold's new book "Let Food Be Your Medicine" aims to shed light on the importance of a healthy diet and its profound impact on our lives. It underscores the significance of nurturing our bodies with nutritious choices and emphasizes the transformative power that food can have on preventing and treating various diseases. His book is a guide to help you choose the right foods, and how you can live a disease-free life, relying solely on the healing properties of the food on our plates.

This book explores in depth the scientifically supported evidence highlighting the link between diet and health. It offers practical and easy-to-implement guidelines for incorporating healthier eating habits into our daily lives. Moreover, "Let Food Be Your Medicine" presents an integrated approach to dietary changes, providing insights into the overall impact on mental and physical well-being. A sure to be a Best Seller

DR. ERIC KAPLAN D.C.,
FIAMA, 5-time #1 Bestselling author.

* * *

Dr. Steven Kringold is a doctor on a mission! He is passionately devoted to reinventing healthcare and reversing chronic disease by promoting healthy foods as our primary 'farmacy' of life. His functional medicine approach promises to hold the keys to lifelong vitality and wellbeing. Count me IN!

ANN LOUISE GITTLEMAN, PHD, CNS

Multi-award-winning NY TIMES bestselling author of more than 35 books
Author of national bestseller <u>Radical Metabolism</u> and <u>Radical Longevity</u>

***

In today's overwhelming sea of health advice, Let Food Be Your Medicine stands out as a much needed and refreshing resource. Dr. Steve's expertise combined with his compassionate tone make this book not only informative but also genuinely empowering, encouraging readers to take charge of their own health in a meaningful and sustainable way. If you're looking for a game-changing read that blends medical authority with a holistic perspective, this is the book to pick up!"

DR EMEE VIDA ESTACIO,
Health Psychologist and Founder of The PAME Code

***

This is a well thought out guide for a healthy diet no matter who or what age you are. The book is not only educational, but also packed with extensively researched historical and up-to-date information for a meaningful lifestyle. Dr. Steve has a knack of lightening and simplifying an otherwise serious topic with his ability to connect personally, experientially, and humorously. It is a rare and refreshing to find a doctor who tells it as it is from a pharmaceutical and "farm"aceutical perspective

Let Food Be Your Medicine is an eye-opener and a must read for anyone who wants not only to age well but to have a wonderful quality and outlook during their adventure on Earth. This book is a practical guide for a healthier life and is full of additional resources. It's a shame we aren't taught at an early age these basic skills and understandings of how to manage our bodies, known as the temple, where our consciousness resides. When I came to the last period in this book, I closed it with a feeling of inspiration and empowerment. That's what the good doctor wants to share. He wants everyone to take back control of their lives through diet to manage aging, disease, weight gain, cognition; and to live life in a more positive and meaningful way.

JACKIE EDGINGTON,
Yoga teacher

***

"Let Food Be Your Medicine" is an excellent and well documented handbook on the link between nutrition and disease and how a highly processed diet can contribute to diseases and a very healthy diet primarily consists of fruits and vegetables can help prevent and often bring us back to health. We are what we eat. This book offers excellent and pertinent information on how to improve our health. It underscores the significance of nurturing our bodies with nutritious choices and emphasizes the transformative power that food can have on preventing and treating various diseases. By choosing the right foods, we can live a disease-free life, relying solely on the healing properties of the food on our plates.

Dr. Steve Kringold, specializes in anti-aging medicine and offers well documented practical guidelines that are easy to incorporate into our lifestyle to live the healthiest life we can. The lists of foods for different diseases serve as an excellent shopping list for health. I learned so much from reading this book and highly recommend it.

BARBARA ZERETSKY,
Runner and Health Enthusiast

LET FOOD BE YOUR MEDICINE

DR. STEVE'S GUIDE TO MANAGE YOUR HEALTH, AGING, DISEASE, AND WEIGHT GAIN

BY DR. STEVE KRINGOLD

© **Copyright 2023 - All rights reserved.**

The content contained within this book may not be reproduced, duplicated, or transmitted without direct written permission from the author or the publisher.

Under no circumstances will any blame or legal responsibility be held against the publisher, or author, for any damages, reparation, or monetary loss due to the information contained within this book, either directly or indirectly.

Legal Notice:

This book is copyright protected. It is only for personal use. You cannot amend, distribute, sell, use, quote or paraphrase any part, or the content within this book, without the consent of the author or publisher.

Disclaimer Notice:

Please note the information contained within this document is for educational and entertainment purposes only. All effort has been executed to present accurate, up to date, reliable, complete information. No warranties of any kind are declared or implied. Readers acknowledge that the author is not engaged in the rendering of legal, financial, medical, or professional advice. The content within this book has been derived from various sources. Please consult a licensed professional before attempting any techniques outlined in this book.

By reading this document, the reader agrees that under no circumstances is the author responsible for any losses, direct or indirect, that are incurred as a result of the use of the information contained within this document, including, but not limited to, errors, omissions, or inaccuracies.

This book is not meant to be a replacement for nutritional or physical health. It's essential that you seek professional advice from your doctor or dietitian first before following through with the advice within this text.

DEDICATION

This book is dedicated to my wife, Debra. She has been the perfect partner in marriage and life and has been instrumental in helping me beat cancer and getting healthy. One of the reasons I love her so much, is that she reminds me to walk the talk and serves as my compass to stay the path and always practice what I preach.

I also dedicate this book to all my readers, in hopes that it serves as a beacon and guide to improve their health and gives them the reasons to adhere to a healthy lifestyle.

JUST FOR YOU!

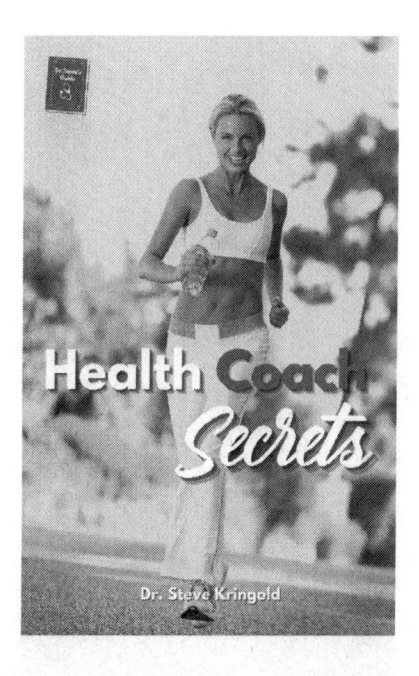

A SPECIAL GIFT FOR OUR READERS

Included with your purchase of this book is a special bonus book I want you to have, which will help you on your journey to Aging Gracefully in the best of health.

Please click the link below to get this important addition.

You'll receive my Health Coach Secrets book which includes:

Diet tips to help you eat clean, an emotional eaters guide, managing food cravings, and chapters on processed foods and grains and sugar detox. You'll also be getting my macronutrients training guide and my 21-day interactive move well program for balance and fitness.

Click the URL below to receive!

https://bit.ly/healthcoachsecrets

ABOUT THE AUTHOR
DR. STEVE KRINGOLD

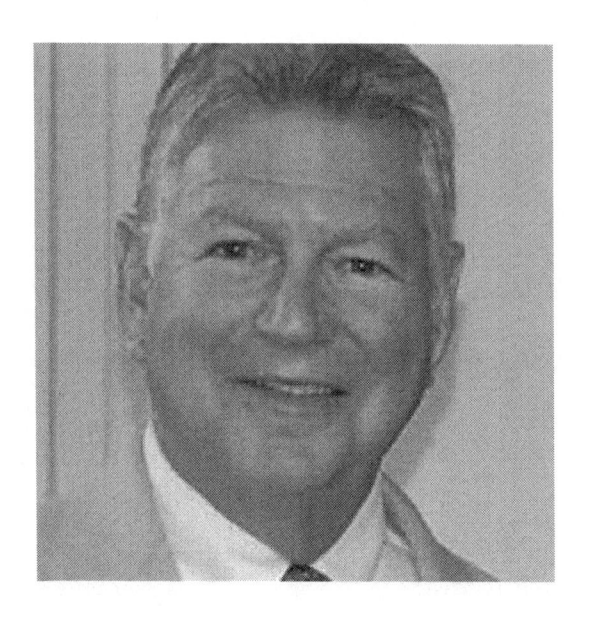

Dr. Steve is a bestselling author and native of South Florida, graduate of Tulane University and the Rosalind Franklin University of Medicine and Science. He is married to Debra, a retired opera singer and currently an artist whose medium has been acrylics and oils, clay, and glass for the past two decades. He has two daughters and 3 grandchildren.

As a member of the American Academy of Anti-Aging Medicine and the American Society of for Nutrition, and through his medical, health and fitness conferences and subscriptions, he stays up to date the latest advances in the anti-aging, health, and fitness genres. He posts daily articles on his Facebook group, "Anti-Aging, Health, and Fitness Community", a group page where members share their thoughts, challenges, and health hacks.

https://www.facebook.com/groups/873179794079005/

Dr. Steve is a former team doctor for the University of Miami Hurricanes and Miami City Ballet, who specialized in sports medicine, foot and ankle surgery, and wound care. He is a certified nutrition coach and member of Healthgrades Consumer Advisory Council. He has completed several marathons, practiced and taught yoga, and eats a healthy diet of mostly fruits and vegetables.

He is a cancer survivor in his 70's and has always been passionate about anti-aging, health, and fitness, with an emphasis on treating patients with a natural approach using diet and exercise. A sought-after lecturer in the health and fitness genre, he has appeared in both masterminds and summits. You can learn more about him by reading his books.

CONTENTS

DEDICATION vii
ABOUT THE AUTHOR ix
INTRODUCTION 1

PART I: THE EVOLUTION OF DIETARY PROBLEMS

CHAPTER 1: Nutritional Nuisance 9
    The Mists of Time 9
    The Sick Diets of Now 17
    Can We Have a Real, Real-Food Diet? 27

CHAPTER 2: Curses of the Modern Life 31
    The Woes of Modern Living 33
    Gut Health 35
    Immune System 39

CHAPTER 3: The Doctor of the Future 43
    Treating Symptoms and Not the Cause 45
    Preventive Medicine 57
    The Body's Ability to Self-Heal 58
    The End of the Beginning 60

PART II: FOOD IS YOUR MEDICINE

CHAPTER 4: The Building Blocks 63
Food as Medicine 63
Nutrition 101 70
Being a Food Sleuth 74
Balancing Your Meals 77
The Functions of Foods 79
Portion Size 83
Beverages 85

CHAPTER 5: Stepping Up Your Nutrition Game .. 87
Vitamins and Minerals 87
Nutrient Deficiencies 94
When to Eat 97
How to Eat 99

CHAPTER 6: What Does Your Gut Say? 105
A Gut Feeling 106
Ground Control to Major Tom 108
The Gut and Immunity 109
Your Gut Health Plan 113
Ambrosia 114
Avoid! Avoid! Avoid! 117
Feeling Pooped? 118

CHAPTER 7: You Only Have to Look Within 123
Eating Your Way to Immunity 125
Your Chemical Romance 131

CHAPTER 8: The Superfoods 139
Just What Is a Superfood? 140
Probiotics 144

Prebiotics 146
Fermented Foods 148
Fiber-Rich Foods 149
Live Long and Prosper 153

PART III: A LIFESTYLE OF CHANGE

CHAPTER 9: Healthy Habits in Motion 161
Building New Habits 162
Beating Cravings 168
Activate Exercise 176

CHAPTER 10: Keep Calm and Carry On 189
Stress!!! 190
Immunity and Stress 198
Taking a Chill Pill 199
Meditation 202
Long-Term Stress Relief 205

CHAPTER 11: Lullaby of a Healthy Life 209
The Science of Sleep 210
Learning to Dance with the Sandman 212

CHAPTER 12: Nature Has the Answer 221
Plants That Heal 223
Garbage Out 227

CONCLUSION 230
APPENDIX A 233
APPENDIX B 243
OTHER BOOKS BY DR. STEVE KRINGOLD 256
REFERENCES 257

> **LET FOOD BE THY MEDICINE AND MEDICINE BE THY FOOD.**
>
> — HIPPOCRATES

INTRODUCTION

There is an often-used acronym in computing circles: GIGO; garbage in, garbage out. In a sense, that is what this book is about. Instead of a computer, it is your body we will be considering. The food you take into your body, not surprisingly, affects how your body works, and it can also damage it. Poor diet is a huge risk factor in many chronic diseases. (Fanelli et al., 2020).

We are always being told what not to eat, things that are bad for us: fatty foods, sugar, and so on. But what about the other side of the coin? Are there foods that are beneficial to us?

We'll talk about this in detail in this book. In the chapters to follow, we will look at how various foods can improve your health and also be used to treat certain conditions. The most obvious is weight control. Being overweight not only reduces the quality of life but can also lead to diseases such as type-2 diabetes. (CDC, n.d.).

This isn't something new. The centrality of diet in our general wellbeing and the use of foods to treat conditions goes way back to the ancient Greeks and, in particular, Hippocrates.

Most people have heard of the Hippocratic oath. What they don't realize is that the original oath in ancient Greek actually refers to food. "With regard to healing the sick, I will devise and order for them the best diet, according to my judgment and means; and I will take care that they suffer no hurt or damage." ("Hippocratic Oath," n.d.). In many translations, the word diet is replaced with medicine.

Like Hippocrates, you will come to realize that the artificial, modern separation of food from pharmaceutical medicines is false. We all tend to see foods as being necessary for growth and energy, and we miss out completely on their medicinal nature.

Hippocratic dietetics was based on observation, much in the same way that soldiers knew that if the arrow didn't kill you, the probable infection would. The scientific explanations the ancients devised to explain their observations were mostly wide of the mark at best. (Moncorgé, n.d.). However, that does not undermine the observations that eating such and such food helped or cured a particular ailment.

It is this natural observation of cause and effect that is missing from our rigid separation of food from medicines. When people talk about food being medicines, there is a tendency to insert the word "like" before medicine. Yet foods are not "like" medicines.

They *are* medicines.

Today, we have a bewildering array of modern medicines that help us fight disease. However, food is unquestionably the first line of defense against disease. At the risk of a terrible pun, why use a sledgehammer to crack a nut? (More about nuts later). If you have a good diet, then the nutrients you are ingesting will be doing the

INTRODUCTION

job of fighting ailments and reducing your risk of a range of severe diseases in a completely natural way.

When was the last time you looked at the leaflet that comes with medicines? Do I need to mention side-effects? Like the sledgehammer, powerful medicines can cause damage as well as mitigate a disease.

If you can reduce the risk or even fight disease by eating well, then you will be less likely to face the risks associated with pharmaceuticals.

It might surprise you to know that poor diet is the leading cause of death in the US. The dietary risk, including body, mass, and index (BMI) and other factors, is almost half of all risks, almost two and a half times that for tobacco. In 2012, poor diet contributed to nearly 1.4 million American deaths. Worse still is that almost half of Americans are living with diet-related illnesses and two-thirds of the population are classed as obese. (CDC, n.d.). The following are just some of the conditions associated with poor diet (Ajmera, 2009):

- Obesity
- Hypertension
- High cholesterol
- Heart disease
- Diabetes
- Stroke
- Gout
- Cancer

You might find yourself taking expensive medicines and therapies to deal with conditions that are entirely due to what you eat and what you are not eating.

If you want to lose weight, feel younger and full of energy, extend your lifespan, reduce your risk of serious disease, reduce your risk of age-related disease, and improve your overall health, then the answer is right in front of you on your plate!

Getting healthier through a good diet isn't just about your body and how it feels. You will also feel a change in your mental state too. As we will see later, your brain actually needs certain types of fats to stay healthy. ("Diet and Mental Health," 2022).

Your confidence will increase. You will be less prone to depression, fatigue, and irritability. Even better, fewer people will swipe left when they see you (on a dating app or in person!) Who doesn't want to look gorgeous?

Maybe you won't have to spend as much on clothes and hair dressing. Like the Fonz, you'll take one look in the mirror and recognize you are at your peak.

You are reading this book probably because you are at a point where you realize that symptom-relieving medicines, fad diets, and expensive therapies aren't making the difference you need. You have come to the GIGO conclusion.

You know, deep down, that you need to make a fundamental change in what you put into your mouth in order to make that switch from coping with poor health to enjoying the freedom of a body and mind that is getting the right balance of nutrients.

You realize that our modern diets have strayed away from the path of wholesome, nutritious foods into the dark forest of processed, unhealthy alternatives. We know there are dangerous things

INTRODUCTION

lurking, but we can't see them, and we often don't know they are there until it's too late.

So, like a good horror movie where the golden rule should always be, "Don't split up," our words of power should be, "don't eat junk!"

You may also have realized that you are eating too many processed foods and ready-made meals because you have a hurried lifestyle that leads you to take the path of least resistance. In addition to changing what you eat, you now want to change your approach to food, making it central to your regime of well-being.

This change in lifestyle, focusing on what really matters, will not only help with your physical health but also with your sleep routine and stress levels—something you know you have been ignoring because stress is just part of modern life. But like bad eating habits, stress doesn't need to be such a negative part of life.

I'm one of those people that practices what I preach. Throughout my many years in the practice of medicine and foot and ankle surgery, I have not only helped everyone from individual patients to the University of Miami's athletic department and Miami City Ballet improve their lifestyles and eating habits, but I have also helped myself enjoy life to its fullest—everything from beating cancer to running marathons. Mind you, as a happily married man and at my stage in life, I'm not bothered if I get swiped left.

It was that close shave with cancer that really made me double down on maintaining a healthy lifestyle and see that food is the best route to a long and healthy life.

Now, to finish the nitty gritty, what will you gain from this book? Better still, what will you gain as a result of putting into practice the lessons learned? Here is a broad list of ideas:

- A deeper and wider understanding of the role that food plays in good health and fighting disease.
- Knowledge of the medicinal and health-promoting benefits of various food types and specific foods.
- Putting important things, like food, at the center of your life.
- A better and healthier life.
- A longer life.
- A life with less illness.
- Slowing down aging.
- Living a more natural life.
- Improved confidence.
- Better mental health.
- Better gut health.
- Weight loss.

PART I
THE EVOLUTION OF DIETARY PROBLEMS

> **NOTHING IN BIOLOGY MAKES SENSE, EXCEPT IN THE LIGHT OF EVOLUTION.**
>
> — THEODOSIUS DOBZHANSKY

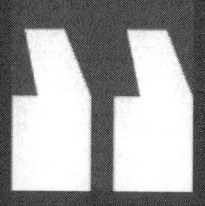

CHAPTER 1:
NUTRITIONAL NUISANCE

The Mists of Time

We all need to eat. It's one of the main commonalities we have as a species. You and I know that our distant ancestors didn't have microwaves and ready-made meals. But what did they eat? How did our eating habits change over the millennia to bring us to where we are now, with a fast-food outlet on every corner?

Early Human Diet

Our most distant ancestors were nomadic hunter-gatherers. They didn't farm; they ate what they found and what they hunted. Their lifestyle followed the seasons, often migrating with their prey or changing their diet to eat what was prevalent in a particular season.

Often, small tribes would exhaust the resources of an area and be forced to move on to places where there was still plenty of food.

You might think, "What a difficult life. Thank goodness we invented farming." It is true that farming brought with it more stability with a regular, if seasonal, supply of food. Not only that, but the density of food production also increased. If we were still hunter-gatherers today, then the food density of the United States would only support 600 thousand people, and the entire planet would only be able to support 10 million. (Paleolithic societies, 2017).

This steady source of food led to population growth. As people were now fixed in one place, villages grew, then towns, cities, nations, and empires.

Farming didn't appear until about 12 thousand years ago (National Geographic Society, 2022), despite our species being around for nearly 200 thousand years. (History.com Editors, 2018). This change probably occurred due to the end of the ice age, which allowed seasonal plants like wild cereals to thrive.

The farm animals we are familiar with today—sheep, goats, pigs, and cattle—were domesticated around the same period in the fertile crescent that covered an area from eastern Turkey down through Iraq to northern Iran.

There was a downside though. Pre-agriculture tribes were more egalitarian, with very little in the way of hierarchy. Famines and droughts were common. Wars started over territory. The more land you controlled, the more people you could feed, and as a result, the richer and more powerful you became.

The really surprising thing, though, is that the general health of humans declined. First, studies of bones, dental cavities and abscesses, and adult height reveal that hunter-gatherers were much taller, had better bone density, less fractures, and much fewer cavities and abscesses. The evidence from skeletons also shows that farming communities had more incidence of diseases than the hunter-gatherer populations. Furthermore, it is clear that most suffered from iron deficiency and delays in development.

I say this is surprising, as up until 1984, it had always been assumed that the introduction of farming would have been beneficial. (Mummert et al., 2011).

Can you guess why health declined with the introduction of farming?

The answer is quite simple. Hunter-gatherers had a very varied diet. As we will see in the rest of this book, variety is not only the spice of life; it is essential to health. The new farming societies became heavily dependent on a limited variety of foods, mainly cereals and meat.

Even today, the global share of calorie intake is dominated by three foods: corn, rice, and wheat, which accounts for 51% of all calories we consume as a species. (Pariona, 2019).

This over-reliance on a very restricted range of food sources is what caused the decline in health at the dawn of agriculture, and it continues to this day.

As you read this, think of the items that make up the bulk of your diet. What variety do you have? Do you regard your diet as wide, or do you have the same breakfast, the same lunch, the same snacks, and the same dinners from day to day and week to week?

There are still tribes around the world that have hunter-gatherer lifestyles, such as the Tsimane of Bolivia and the Hadza of Tanzania. Anthropologists studying these widely distant tribes have discovered that they suffer less from high blood pressure, cardiovascular disease, and atherosclerosis.

In our evolution, meat has been vitally important. Meat is very calorie dense, and we can extract energy from it more easily than from fibrous plants. As our gut shrank in size, our brains grew larger. Our bodies were able to divert more energy to our brains due to this shrinkage. (Gibbons, n.d.).

Recently, there has been a lot of interest in what is known as the paleo diet or caveman diet. The argument is that we should only eat what our bodies were evolved for, and that would be what our distant ancestors dined on, such as meat, fruit, nuts, and some fish.

The diet also advises abstention from grains, beans, and potatoes, as they only appeared with the invention of agriculture.

However, this diet has flaws in its foundations. The first is that anyone who lived in caves did not have the same diet.

A lot depended on the season, the climate, and the part of the world where tribes lived. Even today, when we look at the diets of modern hunter-gatherers, we see a wide variation.

Those that live in tropical climates will mainly eat plants, including tubers and grains. Move into more arctic climes, and the diet shifts to meat and fish. The other reason is that very few people lived to be more than 30. A really old person in paleolithic times would be about 35 years old. Humans back then didn't live long enough for the long-term effects of their diet to kick in. (Coolidge & Wynn, 2013).

If you want to read what hunter-gatherer and agricultural societies were like, including their diet, then read *Stone Spring: The Northland Trilogy*, the science fiction novel by British writer Stephen Baxter. (Baxter, 2012).

The Dawn of Agriculture

Around 10 thousand to 15 thousand years ago, agriculture arose across the globe in places like Africa, the Middle East, China, and South America. This was during a period known as the neolithic or new stone age. It is thought that this step-in civilization came about due to a number of factors.

First, the ice age was ending, and the climate was improving for crops. Humans were now developing much more sophisticated stone tools, which may be due to the evolution of our intellectual abilities, and to round it off, human culture was changing too. It was a Goldilocks moment in our history where everything was "just right."

Something often overlooked though is that a parallel development was taking place, called pastoralism. This occurred in areas where the climate or the terrain wasn't suitable for crops, places that were rocky, for example. Tribes in these areas turned to domesticating and herding animals such as sheep, goats, pigs, and cattle. Bear in mind that these early domesticated animals were quite different from what we see on farms today. Over millennia, selective breeding has transformed these species into creatures that serve our specific needs for wool, milk, and meat.

And with this diversity came trade. Pastoralists would exchange wool, cheese, and other animal products for grains and tubers from agricultural communities. Regrettably, conflict arose between communities too, particularly in the overlap between herding and agricultural communities. (Bergers, 2016). That conflict still continues today. ("Pastoralist and Farmer-Herder Conflicts," 1944).

The impact of agriculture on our world and our species has been immense. Let's just look at some of the effects ("The Dawn of Agriculture," n.d.):

- Greater calorie density per square mile; replacing things we can't eat in a territory with things we can.
- Greater population density due to greater calorie density
- The development of irrigation
- The spread of diseases from close proximity to animals
- Deforestation. We can't eat trees! Farmers, from the earliest times till today, have cleared forests to create more arable land.
- Famine, due to overgrazing, lack of crop rotation, and reduced genetic diversity in crops. The irish potato famine is a good example of when a lack of genetic diversity can wipe out an entire species of plant due to a single disease.
- Reduced diversity in diet
- Trade. Surplus food could be traded for other foodstuffs and items.
- Communal living in towns and cities
- The family unit, property, and inheritance. Now that farmers stayed in one place, they could have larger families, trade wives or daughters, and pass their homes and land down the generations.
- Warfare. Land needed to be defended from invaders, weapons needed to be developed, and towns needed fortifications. The walls of jericho is one example.

- ➢ Division of labor and stratification of society. Now that the land produced more calories, fewer people were needed for food production. At the same time, the population was growing. Now, people could devote their lives to one craft—tanning, building, carpentry, and so on. Society became stratified as trade and property ownership grew.

- ➢ Codified laws, writing, and bureaucracies. In primitive tribes, laws would have revolved around customs set by the seasons, religious beliefs, and taboos. Now that property had come on the market—pun intended—laws had to be agreed to and recorded.

As you can see, it's a mix of good and bad.

If we start by assuming that the birth of agriculture had never occurred, then you wouldn't be reading this book, as writing would never have been invented, and I wouldn't have been able to create the book, as modern technology such as the laptop I am pecking at with my fingers at this very moment wouldn't exist.

Oh, and I would have died 40 years ago. On the plus side, I wouldn't have suffered colon cancer, as I wouldn't have lived long enough for it to develop! Not sure that qualifies as a silver lining.

We have touched briefly on two issues: the paleo diet and selective breeding. Remember: The main thrust of the paleo diet insists that we should only eat what our ancestors ate because that is what we have evolved to eat.

However, one major assumption in that argument is that we have stopped evolving. But we haven't.

Our evolution continues as it does for all species. Gene variants arise all the time. Most of these variants are junk and either do nothing or cause disease. A few, though, are useful.

A simple example of this is how people of European origin have evolved to drink milk. Dairy farming spread into Europe from the Middle East. Before its arrival, Europeans could not properly digest cow's milk. Even today, there are many people who are lactose intolerant. Along the way, a gene variant occurred that permitted lactose tolerance.

This gene became more dominant, as those that have it now have more chances of living than those who don't, primarily because they have access to a food source rich in nutrients.

It isn't quite selective breeding, but choosing dairy farming would have bred out more and more of those who were lactose intolerant. Just comparing

Indigenous North Americans—between 80% to 100% are lactose intolerant and 21% of Anglo Americans are intolerant—highlights how much has changed. In most European countries, intolerance is 15% or less. In Britain, it is somewhere between 5% and 15%. (Lois, 2017).

And this is just milk.

We find the same patterns with other foodstuffs. I suppose this is the ultimate vindication of the old adage, "You are what you eat." A more fitting variation might be, "Your descendants become what you eat."

The Sick Diets of Now

Where Did It All Go Wrong?

Taking as our starting point that pre-agriculture humans were generally healthier and taller than post-agriculture humans, and looking around today at a society that is full of sick, fat, and unhealthy people; we have to ask ourselves, how did it get this bad?

Before we get to answering that, let's look at the startling statistics on what kills us (Rayner, 2018):

- ➢ One billion people suffer from obesity and diabetes.
- ➢ One-third of cancer deaths are diet related.
- ➢ 972 million people are estimated to have high blood pressure (Dobrić, 2020).
- ➢ Nearly 50 million people suffer from dementia.
- ➢ There are more than 80 autoimmune diseases.

Added to this is the psychological harm caused by being unhealthy. People worry and feel shame, guilt, and despair about their physical condition.

All these things lead to poorer quality of life, more illness, and more rapid aging.

I guess that's why you chose to read this book.

Our unhealthy diet has unfolded into two main stages: the introduction of agriculture, narrowing our food sources—and, consequently, our vitamins and minerals—and the development of modern farming methods over the last century into industrial agriculture. (Pratt, 2022).

We Need to Talk About Gluten

Gluten, a problem to many, was introduced with agriculture when we started growing grains in quantity. Gluten and other gluten-like proteins are found in the following:

- Wheat
- Barley
- Rye
- Spelt
- Durum

If you need to avoid gluten, then the best grains are as follows (Pratt, 2022):

- Oats
- Quinoa
- Brown rice
- Corn
- Millet
- Amaranth
- Teft
- Buckwheat

If you actually have a severe allergy to gluten, then you need to be careful to choose grains that are processed in gluten-free conditions to avoid cross-contamination.

The Ultra-Processed Pandemic

We have just experienced the COVID-19 pandemic, and here we are using that word in the context of what is on our plate. Well, in many ways, the processed foods we tend to eat today behave like a virus in a pandemic. Some food-processing methodologies or dietary habits usually start in one place and then spread across the globe.

Take snacking, for example. I can remember my parents constantly telling me not to eat between meals as it would spoil my appetite. It was pretty much the dietary zeitgeist.

Where is that now?

Snacking is now common almost worldwide. It started in countries that were wealthy and had extra money to spend on, well, anything. Those in the food industry realized there was more money to be made so new products were born that would increase our eating opportunities.

As other countries became wealthier, the virus of snacking spread there too. China, for example, did not have a snacking culture. It was only since the millennium that snacking took off. At first, it was what we might term "good" snacks—including fruit and the like. But now, the snacks we all eat in the west are a seven-billion dollar industry.

As you read through this book, you will encounter the Mediterranean diet often. Ironically, the unhealthy snacking and processed food culture is as prevalent there as anywhere else.

The healthiest diets in the world are in the least affluent countries. Chad, Mali, Cameroon, Guyana, Tunisia, Sierra Leone, Laos, Nigeria, Guatemala, and French Guiana top the list of healthiest general diets. (Wilson, 2019).

Don't get me wrong; there is a lot of malnutrition in these countries. Yet that is to do with the scarcity of food rather than its quality.

Processing Sucks the Vitality Out of Foods

Every form of food processing reduces the nutrient value of foods, even good old-fashioned cooking. For example, B and C vitamins are soluble in water, but we often boil vegetables, which leads to these necessary vitamins leaching out of them and into the water—not great unless you are making soup.

That's not to say that cooking is all bad. Plant cells have a thick cell wall. Cooking breaks down this cell wall, releasing the trapped nutrients ready to be absorbed in our digestive tract. It also kills off bacteria (but not toxins produced by bacteria).

Tomatoes are good for you. Cooked tomatoes are even better, as the process releases phytochemicals that are powerful antioxidants.

Cooking has been with us for a very, very long time. Still, other processes have been around for just as long, like fermenting, milling, and preserving with salt or brine. Preserving made food last longer and helped with trading food and dealing with winter. (Park, 2021).

Cooking, fermentation, and milling all help to release nutrients from food. Small beer was drunk by all ages during the middle ages, the content in it usually being less than 1%. However, alcohol is still a toxin—just ask anyone with a hangover. However, its toxicity kills off bacteria (which is the purpose of the alcohol rub you get before an injection). As a result, small beer was safer to drink than water. It was also a source of many nutrients. ("Small Beer," 2001).

On balance, most of this type of processing is good. However, we turn our attention now to the dark side of processing. First, let's look at the purposes of processing ("The Top Boron," n.d.):

- Preserving
- Encouraging the growth of foods
- Killing harmful organisms
- Releasing nutrients
- Flavor enhancing
- Appearance enhancing

Now, looking at that list, you would be forgiven for thinking, "Sounds good to me!" Why would you not want all these amazing things? Let's dig deeper and see what processing actually does to the nutritional content of food ("The Top Boron," n.d.).

- **Fertilizers** encourage plant growth, and so do hormones in animals. In humans, ingested fertilizers can cause cancers, respiratory problems, and heart disease. (Kerkar, 2019). The hormones pumped into animals are consumed by you when you eat animal products. In humans, growth hormones ingested in this way can lead to cancers, sexual disorders, and a decrease in the male-to-female ratio. ("The Environmental and Health Impacts of Growth Hormones," 2013). In fact, many states, including the European Union, have banned the use of growth hormones and the import of meat produced using these hormones. ("Hormones in Meat," n.d.).

- **Blanching** involves heating a food very quickly before freezing, drying, or canning in order to make the color, flavor, and texture last longer. It involves immersion in a hot liquid like boiling water or oil. Unfortunately, water-soluble vitamins like the B-complex and C can be destroyed by blanching.

- **Canning** involves heating the food inside to a very high temperature to kill micro-organisms. Again, the water-soluble vitamins like B-complex and C can be destroyed. ("Food Processing," n.d.).

- **Milling** cereals removes the outer husk and releases the inner nutrients. The husks, however, contain minerals, phytochemicals, and B-complex vitamins.

- **Freezing** is the least damaging process as, usually, the defrosted food is virtually unchanged.

- **High-pressure treatment** kills micro-organisms but retains more of the nutrient content than other processes.

- **Pasteurization** of milk and fruit juices kills micro-organisms without too much loss of nutrient value, although vitamin C can be lost in fruit juices.

- **Drying foods** can reduce the amount of vitamin C at the same time as concentrating other nutrients. This concentration also applies to the calorie per unit volume and could cause obesity.

- **Trimming and peeling** of vegetables often removes a significant amount of nutrients that are just under the skin.

So that's the more traditional type of processing. Next up, is ultra-processing. Yeah, it gets worse.

The Death of Nutrition

Ultra-processing procedures are often much more technical in their nature and involve things like hydrogenation, which is used to make margarine from oil. This actually changes unsaturated fats into saturated fats. There are many other processes, such as fractionation, hydrolysis, pre-frying, extrusion, and molding.

Aside from these processes, this class of foods has many additives, including sugars, salt, fats, oils, artificial flavorings and colors, inverted sugars, flavor enhancers like MSG, and emulsifiers.

These processes and additives take foods as far from natural as it is possible to get. It's no accident that they are often called junk food.

It's probably a good idea to get to know what types of foods are ultra-processed.

- Any powdered foods such as soups, desserts, and noodles.
- Pre-prepared foods such as pasta, meat, pizzas, and cheese dishes.
- Candy.
- Energy drinks and sodas.
- Salty snacks.
- Biscuits and pastries.
- Added sugar breakfast cereals.
- Reconstituted meat products like burgers, sausages, and hot dogs.

Looking at that list, there is probably one word we would associate with them: popular.

They are popular because they are very palatable. They also form the basis of the fast-food business and, with our hurried lifestyles, are convenient. They are also much cheaper than fresh foods.

Just how popular and cheaper? Well, according to recent research, as much as 73% of the American diet is ultra-processed, and those foods are 52% cheaper. (Agostino, 2022).

No wonder we have problems with conditions associated with poor diet. These conditions include the following:

- Cardiovascular diseases
- Metabolic diseases
- Cancer
- Obesity
- Gastrointestinal disorders
- Depression

The four apocalyptic horsemen driving our need to consume such unhealthy products are as follows (Lehman, 2022):

- **Price.** They are very much cheaper than wholesome foods.
- **Flavor.** Salt, sugar, fats, oils, and enhancers are added to give an instant hit. This is what makes these foods so tasty and addictive.
- **Convenience.** They can be stored longer than whole foods and are quick to rustle up a meal or snack.
- **Habit,** which is often overlooked. As much as 70% of what we do every day is habit driven. This includes our eating habits. (Duhigg, 2014).

Ultra-processing destroys the complex structure of plant and animal cells resulting in a mush, which is very low in nutrients, which our bodies can absorb rapidly. (Spector, 2020).

A word of warning to vegans: Your diet is often seen as healthy, but take care with foods that are meant to mimic traditional non-vegan foods such as burgers and dairy products like milk. These are ultra-processed foods with all the bad stuff we have looked at. (Anthony, 2022).

As ultra-processed foods are easy to chew and gulp down, they are faster to eat. This ends up with people eating much more when they are eating mainly ultra-processed foods compared to whole food diets—as much as 500 calories more, according to research. (Servick, 2019).

No Easy Way Out

You are sitting there thinking, "That's it! No more junk food for me!" Smiling, you think the problem is now solved.

Sorry to burst your bubble. Modern farming methods have reduced the nutritional content of our foods. The humble potato now contains 28% less calcium, 57% less vitamin C, and 100% less vitamin A than its distinguished grandfather back in 1950. (Hailey, 2021a).

Often the blame is laid at the door of selective breeding, but a significant factor is the decline in the nutritional content of soil. Almost 99% of our calories originate from the soil. (Melville, 2020). The problem is that inorganic fertilizers with high nitrogen content kill-off microbes in the soil that are central to soil health. The microbes basically make the nutrients for plants. Overtime, if the same soil is mismanaged over and over, the nutrient content of the soil rapidly declines, leading to fewer nutrients in the crops.

The old adage, "You are what you eat," applies just as much to plants as it does to us. Their food is also junk. While we worry about the lack of nutrients in our diet, triffids are just as worried about the lack of nutrients in the soil; maybe that's why they started eating us. Little did they know that we are just as nutrient deficient!

My basil plant outside just isn't doing well, but my wife grows basil in our kitchen, a gathering place in our home. The carbon dioxide we breathe out is why her basil thrives. The growth of plants is built on carbon dioxide; it lets them "breathe" it in and "breathe" out oxygen. We are gas buddies with our plant.

Wait, haven't we heard of carbon dioxide before? It's that nasty greenhouse gas that is causing climate change. It also turns out that, like us, plants can have too much of a good thing. The predicted carbon dioxide levels in 2050 have been shown to lower the levels of protein, zinc, and iron in a range of plants. Some vitamins have been shown to drop by as much as 50%. (Suglia, 2018). Of course, by then, our soil will be even more nutrient deficient than it is now. Everything that we are doing to our environment is conspiring to reduce the nutrients in our food.

Genetically modified organisms (GMOs) are the new kid in town. This is a highly technical intervention in the breeding of plants. It is too early to tell if they are bad for us, as they have only been around for 30 years or so. Unlike new medicines that need to undergo various levels of study before even being trialed on humans, GMOs have found their way into our foods without much research to see if they cause any harm. (Hailey, 2021b).

The main problem with GMOs is that the modifications to the plant's DNA are almost always for one purpose: to increase production. This is achieved by using gene inserts in the plant's DNA to improve higher tolerance of herbicides, pest resistance (Bt Corn is genetically modified to produce the insecticide Bt toxin, for example), virus resistance, and metabolic shifts such as preventing apples from browning when they are cut.

Whether or not GMOs turn out to be harmful, they are encouraging greater and greater use of monoculture farming where the same vast areas are framed with the same crop, year after year, degrading the nutrient content of the soil.

Eating whole foods is a step in the right direction. Unfortunately, the end zone has been moved due to the decline of soil nutrients and we can't produce the same quantities of crops as before.

<u>Nutrient Measuring</u>

One way of measuring a plant's nutrients is to take a Brix reading using a refractometer. It measures the sugar sap content of a plant. The higher the reading, the healthier the plant and the better for us in terms of nutrients. This greater density of nutrients also comes with better flavor.

Can We Have a Real, Real-Food Diet?

Without a major change in farming methods, the answer is no. As we have seen, the actual nutrient value of the soil is declining dramatically. At the same time, more processes are used in the farming, processing, and storage of whole foods.

Apples can be sprayed with up to 42 pesticides. Last night, I had a lovely salmon carpaccio with avocado and shallots. Healthy, right? However, it was farmed salmon. As much as 90% of U.S. consumption of salmon is farmed. ("Why Real Food Is No Longer Enough," 2016).

Then there is the plastic we eat. Oh yes, we do. If you choose foods wrapped in plastics, even fresh foods like meat and vegetables, or if you eat canned foods (with a plastic lining), then there is a good chance that you are consuming bisphenol A (BPA). This is an artificial estrogen.

As much as 93% of Americans have this chemical in their bodies. ("How Much Plastic Are You Really Eating", n.d.). Just how bad is BPA? It

- Increases the number of fat cells
- Slows the ability to burn calories
- Affects your perception of hunger
- Possibly develops adhd
- Causes reproductive, immunity, and neurological problems
- Induces a greater risk of alzheimer's
- Can cause childhood asthma, metabolic disease, type 2 diabetes, and cardiovascular disease

Try to avoid using plastic containers, even for reusable drinks. Also, just don't microwave in plastic! As far as possible, purchase foods that aren't plastic wrapped.

Things are changing with plastics, though. More plastics are being made from organic sources. In some parts of Indonesia, beverages are now being sold in edible plastic cups made from seaweed.

Forget the carbs and the fats (not completely though, as we will see later); the most dangerous aspect of modern diets is the deficiency in micronutrients—the vitamins and minerals. This deficiency is the major cause of many diseases.

Changing to a diet rich in micronutrients will not only help prevent numerous health problems, but it will reduce the aging rate of your cells. (Seow, 2023). Your biological age will be younger than it would otherwise be.

A good diet is vital to good health. However, it is only the string section of the orchestra of lifestyle factors that affect your health. In the next chapter, we will look at the woodwind, brass, and percussion sections. Once you have all the instruments performing perfectly, your body will be a symphony of health, maybe the Pastoral Symphony? (Oh dear).

> **THENCEFORTH, EVIL BECAME MY GOOD.**
>
> — MARY WOLLSTONECRAFT SHELLEY

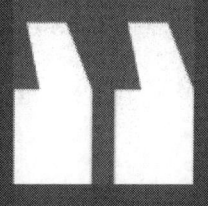

CHAPTER 2:
CURSES OF THE MODERN LIFE

It isn't just bad diets that are killing us. There are many aspects of modern life that are awful. One of these is addiction. Even food can be addictive. If you eat a lot of junk food, then your brain will release dopamine, making you feel wonderful. On top of that, lots of fats and sugars actually increase the receptors in your brain associated with addiction. This is where, like the creature in *Frankenstein*, you will choose a path where "Thenceforth, evil [becomes your] good." (Shelley, 1818).

In the previous chapter, we looked at various diseases that are associated with ultra-processed foods, but they also increase the occurrence of heartburn, which can lead to disease of the esophagus.

Your blood sugar will spike after eating high sugar-content foods. Too much of this, and you are on the road to type-2 diabetes. Your poor kidneys will also suffer due to the high sodium content, sugar, and additives that need to be filtered from your blood.

Your gut isn't just a digestive tube; it contains an ecosystem of microbes that are good for your health. Eating a lot of junk food is equivalent to napalming this diverse community of life in your intestines, possibly leading to gut inflammation and disease of the intestine.

All those fats and sugars can strain your liver and possibly lead to non-alcoholic fatty liver disease (NAFLD).

Want to lose your eyesight by developing age-related macular degeneration (AMD)? Great! Just keep stuffing in those ultra-processed foods. (Alexander, 2023).

Here is a short list of just some of the effects these foods have on you (EcoWatch, 2016 & Brown, 2021):

- Obesity
- Metabolic syndrome
- Inflammatory bowel disease
- Autoimmune diseases
- Colorectal cancer
- Anxiety (since junk food triggers adrenaline release) and depression due to your brain not receiving the hit you get when you eat high sugar-content foods. This also leads to addiction.
- Poor nourishment
- Leaky gut. Partially digested food enters the bloodstream, triggering an immune system response that, overtime, weakens the immune system.

- ➤ Yeast infections. They tire out your immune system, making other infections more likely.
- ➤ Additives, which can also trigger an immune response leading to yet more weakening of the immune system.
- ➤ Wrinkles and sagging skin due to sugars and highly refined grains. Your skin loses elasticity.
- ➤ Acne and other skin conditions can be made worse due to inflammation
- ➤ Poor memory function due to loss of gut microbes
- ➤ Insulin resistance due to high blood sugar, leading to type 2 diabetes, heart disease, and polycystic ovarian syndrome

The Woes of Modern Living

Let's get back to the orchestra we left in chapter one. Let's add in a few more instruments and keep the string section of diet in for completeness. (Farhud, 2015).

- ➤ **Diet** (our string section) and body mass index (BMI) are the most important factors in your health, which is why this book is so focused on this aspect.
- ➤ **Exercise.** Staying active and making sure you have enough exercise improves both your physical and mental health.
- ➤ **Sedentary lifestyle.** Ironically, I am preaching about this as I sit at my desk writing this book. I have a standing desk ordered, so that will help. Today we spend far too much time sitting down, both at work and at leisure. Many jobs are now office based. Fortunately, many companies now

realize the detrimental effect sitting all day has on our health and are now providing standing desks for their employees.

- **Sleep.** Poor sleep patterns and not enough sleep affects your mental and physical health.
- **Sex.** Dysfunctional sex is a vicious circle. Sometimes we find that we can't have normal sexual relations due to either physical or psychological issues. This causes anxiety that then leads to more dysfunction, and round it goes. Counseling can help break loops like this. Of course, risky sex can also lead to sexually transmitted diseases.
- **Substance abuse.** All those hip and not-so-hip illegal drugs come with addiction issues and a range of physical and psychological ailments.
- **Smoking.** Well, you knew that would be here. It's a killer with more than one MO.
- **Alcohol.** Another of the bête noires of life—not that this is modern in any way. Alcohol abuse has been around since the first person learned how to ferment. It is a toxin; it kills bacteria and other organisms. It doesn't do our body much good either and is particularly harmful to the brain, liver, and kidneys. We all have to be careful about our alcohol intake.
- **Prescription drug abuse.** Modern medicine is wonderful, and if it wasn't for all those wonder drugs, half of us (metaphorically speaking; this is not an empirical fact) would be dead. There is a downside, though, if we develop a reliance on them. We enter that brave new world where a gram is better than a damn. We develop a psychological dependency and with many long-term drugs, there are a myriad of health-

damaging side effects. Of course, with some conditions, there is no alternative to taking long-term medication; just ask Kay Redfield Jamison. (Jamison, 2009). She is an American bipolar disorder researcher investigating a condition she has had since early adulthood.

- **Modern technology.** Many of us now spend a significant part of our lives sitting in front of screens either for work or leisure. Overuse may affect sleep patterns, and there is some evidence that mobile phone overuse can cause depression. (Thomée et al., 2011).

- **Recreation.** Just taking time to enjoy pastimes, hobbies, sports, and cultural activities is a good way of relieving stress from our lives.

- **Intellectual pursuits.** Studying new topics, developing new skills, playing games, and good old reading and writing can delay the onset of Alzheimer's by five years. (Lennon, 2021).

It's no secret that, in general, we have too little exercise, too much stress, and too little sleep.

Gut Health

In days gone by, they used to say that you can judge the character of a man by his shoes. In a similar way, we can get a pretty good measure of the quality of our health by looking at the health of our gut.

I have mentioned before that the gut is like an ecosystem of microbes. There are literally trillions of microbes living in our gut, maybe as many as 400 trillion, and as many as 1,000 different species. (Holmes, 2016). Many of these critters are good for our health. They help us to break down foods, provide energy for the gut, make vitamins, neutralize toxins, and fight off pathogens. The presence of these from the moment we are born helps our immune system to develop and to distinguish between good microbes and bad ones.

Nuking these microbes with ultra-processed foods, taking antibiotics when we don't need them, and being too hygienic have resulted in a decline in the populations and varieties of health-promoting microbes in our gut.

In one study, mice were split into two groups. Half were given gut bacteria from lean women and the other half from obese women. These mice, that started off looking identical, quickly diverged. The obese recipients became obese and the others stayed lean and healthy. Both groups were given the same diet in the same amounts. In the second phase, the two groups were mixed together. As a result of probably eating each other's poo, the obese mice acquired the bacteria of the lean mice. Result? The obese mice became leaner. (Owens, 2013).

The initial batch of microbes we receive is from our mother's birth canal. Most of these microbes are symbiotes, meaning that they benefit from us, and we benefit from them. (MacGill, 2023).

In our diets, we should not only consider feeding our health but also the health of the community of microbes that live within us. Keeping them healthy keeps us healthy.

The reduction in our gut bacteria from the natural levels we should have is a major factor in food allergies. Research on the microbiome of people from different cultures shows that there is a significant difference between people in industrialized societies and those living

CURSES OF THE MODERN LIFE

traditional lifestyles. For example, hunter-gathers in Tanzania have more gut microbes that digest plant polysaccharides than those in the industrialized west. This richness of that type of bacteria is indicative of a high-fiber diet. (Guglielmi, 2019).

Some tribes in Papua New Guinea have an extra 50 bacterial types in their gut compared to Americans. (Collyer-Smith, 2015).

There are many factors that contribute to the reduction of the biota in our gut, including the following (Robertson, 2019 & "8 Lifestyle Habits," 2021):

- ➢ Cesarean delivery
- ➢ Antibiotic use. We do need to take antibiotics when we have infections. However, antibiotics not only kill the infection, but they also kill the bacteria in our gut. It can take up to two years for the bacteria to recover. In fact, we're usually prescribed antibiotics when we don't really need them.
- ➢ Smoking. The huge range of harmful chemicals in tobacco smoke harms the gut and the bacteria living there in a variety of ways.
- ➢ Alcohol. As mentioned before, alcohol is a toxin. Fermentation in brewing halts when the alcohol, produced by the yeast as it consumes sugar, reaches a level that kills the yeast. Alcohol kills gut bacteria.
- ➢ Reduced exposure to microbes in early childhood
- ➢ High fat/low carb diet
- ➢ Refined carbohydrates
- ➢ Chemicals such as triclosan (an antibacterial) and parabens (a preservative used in body products)

- ➢ Formula feeding, which plays an important role in establishing a good gut biota in infants
- ➢ Lack of sleep. Keep your sleep pattern to a routine. Not getting enough sleep can harm your gut bacteria and lead to an increase in the bacteria associated with the development of type 2 diabetes and weight gain. (smith et al., 2019).
- ➢ Stress. Stress leads to a decrease in gut bacteria, which can lead to gut inflammation.
- ➢ Lack of diversity in foods. A diet rich in whole foods leads to diverse gut flora.
- ➢ Lack of physical activity. Professional athletes have a more diverse and rich gut biome. Exercise has been shown in many studies to increase the diversity of gut bacteria. (carter et al., 2019).
- ➢ Lack of prebiotics in our diets. This is a type of fiber that we don't digest, but it feeds the microbes in our gut, helping them to thrive and benefit us.

A diet rich in nutrients, especially vitamins C, E, and A, zinc, omega-3 fatty acids, and beta-carotene ameliorates food allergies. On the other side of the coin, eating refined carbs, gluten, omega-6 fatty acids, and lots of additives exacerbate food allergies. (Kresser, 2017).

We often think of our gut as the place where we digest food and give little thought to the role that it plays in our health. But maintaining a healthy gut is essential to promoting overall health. A significant part of that is ensuring, through good whole food and a varied diet rich in micronutrients, our band of bacterial workers are kept happy and healthy.

Immune System

Our bodies are really good at fighting off infection. The immune system is a well-oiled machine crafted by millions of years of evolution.

The creatures that didn't have good immune systems died from infections, and the ones that did survived. Generation after generation, this natural selection of the fittest immune systems has led to the creation of a complex mechanism with many parts serving a variety of roles in keeping us healthy.

If we hadn't invented vaccines for COVID-19, then thousands and thousands of people would have died.

The people left, however, would be the ones that had some sort of immune response that aided their survival.

Overtime, this winnowing of the population would have led to our species evolving to have very good immune systems for fighting the virus.

Like any complex mechanism, it needs to be maintained to keep working properly. Even worse, some of our lifestyle and diet choices can throw a spanner in the works.

In the story so far, we have seen that our modern lifestyle has altered aspects of our bodies. In the last chapter, we looked at how our lifestyles and diets have badly damaged the diversity of our gut microbiome.

This has played a part in wearing down our immune systems and increasing our susceptibility to a wide range of diseases.

Many of the things that we covered earlier in this chapter also weaken the immune system, but it is worth revisiting them again (Premier Wellness Centers, 2020):

- ➢ **Diet.** Too much sugar, pesticides, processed foods, and too much food! There are not enough whole foods and micronutrients in our body.
- ➢ **Toxins** including pesticides, herbicides, molds in old buildings, and exposure to and ingesting heavy metals.
- ➢ **Antibiotics.** 70% of our immune system is in our gut. As we have seen, antibiotics can kill off good gut bacteria.
- ➢ **Not enough exercise.**
- ➢ **Stress,** which can cause depression but also release cortisol, making us more susceptible to viruses.
- ➢ **Not enough sun.** Not only does sunlight produce vitamin D, which is important for our immune system, but it also makes our T cells move faster. T cells are a type of white blood cell that are killer cells that hunt and kill pathogens. ("Sunlight Offers Surprise Benefit," 2016).
- ➢ **Sleep.** When we sleep, our bodies release cytokines needed for the regulation of the immune system. In addition, good sleep boosts the effectiveness of T cells.

As a result of our hurried, stressful, sleep-deprived, exercise-deficient, and poor diet lifestyles, we are much more susceptible to disease than ever before. Ironically, this leads to a greater need for antibiotics, which, in turn, damage particularly the immune-helping bacteria in our gut—a vicious circle.

Our weakened immune systems reduce our expected lifespan through comorbidities. Again, harking back to COVID-19, the people most likely to die were those with weakened immune systems due to comorbidities such as cancer, heart disease, respiratory ailments, depression, and other infections like influenza. These conditions all have a link to poor diet.

Let's look at an example of how diet affects our immune system. The bacteria living in your gut is responsible for fermenting your dietary fiber. This produces short-chain fatty acids, which have a significant role to play in the immune system's fight against cancer, allergies, and autoimmune disease. Just ensuring that you have plenty of fiber in your diet assists the immune system. It's like a bucket brigade fighting a fire. You eat the fiber, the microbes produce the fatty acids, and the immune system utilizes these to fight infection. (Macia et al., 2021). If the first step isn't there, then the rest can't follow.

Stress and sleep are interrelated. As much as 75% of Americans experience moderate to high levels of stress. ("Five Factors," 2021). Stress affects our ability to sleep, either preventing sleep or disrupting our sleep patterns. As a result, we have lower levels of cytokines and are, therefore, more susceptible to infection. We will see in later chapters just how important stress and sleep are in our overall health.

Our gut instinct (Oh dear!) when we are in poor health is to summon the doctor (Okay, I know that doesn't really happen now) or reach for the pills.

We have touched on how making too much use of modern medicine can be detrimental to us. In the next chapter, we will do a deep dive into this.

> **I'M THE DOCTOR, AND I SAVE PEOPLE.**
>
> — DOCTOR WHO

CHAPTER 3:
THE DOCTOR OF THE FUTURE

Doctor Who has lived for 900 years due to a tremendously good diet. FACT! Come on, you didn't really believe that this guy is real, did you?

In this chapter, we will look at modern medicine and how we are not using enough food solutions to promote health, alleviate conditions, and cure ailments.

A colleague of mine has osteoarthritis in his left hand. The doctor he attended prescribed a topical painkiller cream. When his condition worsens, the doctor will probably prescribe anti-inflammatory drugs, which come with the added bonus of potential stomach ulcers, gastrointestinal problems, high blood pressure, cardiovascular disease, and kidney disease.

During the consultation, my good friend mentioned turmeric several times. Not once did the doctor pick up on this or suggest that turmeric in my friend's diet would help.

On another visit for another condition, he brought up the osteoarthritis and turmeric again with another doctor, and this time, no response, again!

Yet many studies have shown that curcumin in turmeric reduces pain significantly. ("7 Health Benefits of Turmeric," 2021). It is well known that it has anti-inflammatory properties. Curcumin reduces the activity of the enzyme COX-2, which is responsible for inflammation and pain. It also changes other pro-inflammatory mechanisms, reducing inflammation. Like anything, there are some side effects to ingesting a lot of turmeric, but they are mild in comparison to modern medicines. (Erickson, 2021).

In general, doctors are not that great at prescribing dietary solutions unless you are obese, where the condition is obviously related to diet.

If you have hypertension, for example, then you will be advised to reduce your salt intake.

However, mostly, any dietary advice is an adjunct to a modern medicine solution and not an alternative.

As we work through this chapter, we will first look at how modern medicine is focused on treating symptoms rather than causes and finish by starting our look at how food can be your medicine.

Our chapter title could do with changing.

The doctor of the future is the doctor of the past. Specifically, good old Hippocrates, who said, "Let food be your medicine."

Treating Symptoms and Not the Cause

I am reminded of a line from a song in the Rocky Horror Picture Show, "So, I'll remove the cause but not the symptom." (Hartley & O'Brien, 1973).

Causation is a topic that has occupied scientists and philosophers for millennia, going right back to Aristotle. (Falcon, 2006). It is clear that everything we see happening around us has a cause—something that made it happen. Yet in the field of medicine and, in particular, the design and production of medicines, the focus is mainly on the treatment of symptoms rather than the cause of those symptoms.

Cynically, we might attribute this to pharma companies not being too interested in actually ridding us of the causes of ailments, as that would mean we wouldn't need an ongoing, often lifelong, supply of drugs to ease the symptoms.

Now, I'm not in the business of denigrating the valuable use of medicines in treatments. I'm not a snake-oil salesman nor a prophet of some new age wonder cure. In my long career in medicine, I have used modern medicines as much as the next doctor. However, during my career, it became increasingly obvious to me that many of the problems we were treating were caused or exacerbated by modern diets.

We are not throwing the baby out with the bath water. The wonderful aids that we have in medicine have improved lives and saved many. What we will be looking at is the role a good diet plays in the armory of weapons we have for fighting disease and making our lives better.

To extend that war metaphor, is it not better to prevent a battle instead of fighting it? Churchill had the same idea when he said, "Better jaw-jaw than war-war." (Meyer, 2012). Food can reduce our need for medicines.

Thomas Edison said, "The doctor of the future will give no medicine, but will interest his patient in the care of the human frame, in diet and in the cause and prevention of disease." ("The Doctor of the Future," 2017). This was before the discovery of Penicillin by the great Scottish scientist Alexander Fleming in 1928 by the way. Now, while Edison may not have envisaged the advances modern medicine would bring, he did hit on the importance of diet and, even back then, the practice of treating symptoms with medicines.

The Failure of Modern Medicine

Changing Medical Practice

Here's a claim that might surprise you: Prescription drugs are the third largest cause of death among Europeans and Americans after cancer and heart disease. (Gøtzsche et al., 2013). There are now dozens of books and papers making similar claims.

Why is such a dramatic claim being made?

My grandfather only sought medical help when he was ill. In general, in his day, people rarely went to the doctor unless they had an obvious infection.

Things have changed since then in two main vaccinations have eliminated a lot of the good diseases that would require a trip to the doctor. Second, we along to our doctor for routine checkups. It's a bit like the MOT test that cars in the UK have to undergo every year to see if they are roadworthy. During these tests, little things are often diagnosed that need treatment.

One of my friends in the UK recently told me that there is a widespread belief that it is in a garage's interest to "find" problems that need fixing, at a sizable cost. Indeed, there is evidence that mechanics will try to sell more repairs to women than men due to a widely held view that men know more about cars. (Banks, 2015).

Aside from bias and naked self-interest, there is a tendency among mechanics, doctors, and other professionals to find things that may only be mild or temporary and assign them a degree of severity beyond what actually exists. This confirmation bias arises as a result of the setting of a diagnosis.

Who goes to a doctor? Who does a doctor treat?

Sick people!

In examination and diagnosis, a doctor is more likely to lend greater weight to any signs he detects that indicate what he expects to see: illness.

Confirmation bias is well understood in science, and scientific research is built around eliminating it using techniques like double-blind tests. Unfortunately, confirmation bias gets more embedded the older we get.

Yet, this isn't the only type of bias that doctors are prone to. There's also (Elston, 2019):

- Anchoring bias: being influenced by initial data. So, don't cough unnecessarily as you enter the doctor's office, even if it's just to clear your throat.

- Availability bias: where the disease that first comes to mind is the most likely. An example of this is a friend who was diagnosed and treated for years for IBS when, in fact, he had helicobacter pylori—a condition easily identified or eliminated by a simple saliva test. It is also treated very simply, with a success rate of around 90%. (De Francesco et al., 2021).

- Premature closure: where the doctor just loves their diagnosis and looks no further.

- Response bias: basing a diagnosis on responses from the patient that may not be accurate. "When do you experience the pain?" the doctor may ask, and the patient responds, "When I've been sitting down for half an hour." However, the doctor has not enquired further to discover that the sitting down is at the dinner table with a plate filled with ultra-processed food. The response from the patient has given a misleading cognitive path for the doctor.

- Framing effect: otherwise known as leading questions. A classic example of this is research into eyewitness testimony, where observers of a car collision were more likely to report broken glass if the word "smash" is used when being questioned. (Yogi, 2016).

- ➢ Omission bias: where the doctor is more likely to choose an option that requires minimal or no intervention. It is easier to choose not to do something than to do it. In one study, doctors were less likely to prescribe when there was a choice between two medicines than when only one medicine was available. (Redelmeier & Shafir, 1995).
- ➢ Overconfidence: a self-belief that their judgment is correct that may not tally with the facts.
- ➢ Sunk cost bias: the gambler's option. Once a track has been chosen and a lot has been invested in that diagnosis, it is difficult to reject it when new evidence arises. Like the gambler, we keep betting on black.

Overdiagnosis and Overtreatment

So, with all this going on, it is little wonder that doctors tend to over diagnose and overtreat their patients. It's the doctor's job to find out what's wrong with you. Take ADHD in children, for example. Many kids across America are prescribed powerful drugs to control their behavior when, in fact, sometimes it is just young children behaving like young children. (Villines, 2021). Have a go at working out how many of the biases above could be at work in this sort of diagnosis.

Side Effects

We all know that drugs have "side effects," but let's be honest, there is nothing sidey about them. They are effects; plain and simple. In other words, the drug does more to your body than its headline act. With many drugs, these effects make you unwell and also kill you.

About 300,000 people die each year in Europe and America due to the "side effects" of prescription drugs. (Light, 2014).

Kill or cure, as the saying goes.

Clinical Trials

Clinical trials come at the end of a long process of testing new drugs in a variety of ways before they get to use them on humans. The objective of a clinical trial is to determine the following:

1. Are the drugs safe?
2. Are they effective?
3. Are they more effective than existing treatments or have fewer side effects?
4. Are there any side effects overtime? This is assessed after the drugs are approved for long-term use over years and decades. In other words, doctors have no idea what the long-term side effects will be when they are prescribing a new drug.

However, phase 4 above is open-ended. Some of the most widely prescribed drugs in America are antidepressants. If they are taken over a long period of time, which they usually are, then the possible side effects include the following (Dellwo, 2022):

- Emotional detachment (65%)
- Sexual problems (72%)
- Increased weight (65%)
- Reduced positivity (46%)
- Suicidal thoughts (36%)
- Not feeling like themselves (54%)

- ➢ Feeling addicted (43%)
- ➢ Caring less about others (36%)

As you can see with those percentages, it's disingenuous to label these as "side" effects, especially in the cases where most people end up suffering from them. The other thing to take from this is that individuals will suffer several of these effects.

Another effect that is usually identified after trials is bad interactions with other drugs and foods. Clinical trials will pick up on some of these, but there is a huge difference between the data collected from a few thousand people during trials and the data that becomes available after people start using them in their millions.

Drugs aren't always trialed on people with the actual conditions the drug is meant to treat; children, pregnant women, and older people are just a few examples. Perhaps the most famous example of this was thalidomide. It wasn't trialed on pregnant women. However, when it was launched after clinical trials on other people, it was marketed as a drug to prevent morning sickness resulting in babies being born with terrible deformities.

Responsibility and Blame

The "Big Pharma" companies are run on the basis of providing a good return to shareholders. They are generally run by individuals with little or no scientific background. They are business professionals. Go back a few decades, and scientists would have been on the board or even running the companies.

It might shock you to know that American doctors accept money and gifts to the tune of $2 billion. (Mitchell & Korenstein, 2020).

Just think, aside from all the biases mentioned above, what other bias might a doctor have for prescribing a particular drug? Their mortgage payments, perhaps?

The gifts range from free meals to luxury destination travel as paid consultants. No less than 36 studies have shown that payments from drug companies affect prescribing. (Mitchell et al., 2021).

When a drug goes badly wrong through overprescribing, misprescribing, or proves to have disastrous effects, then the "Big Pharma" companies are often taken to court where they will vigorously defend their position that the drug did not cause the problems claimed.

After—and often it's after years of litigation—companies can end up paying out billions in fines and compensation if they are found liable. But here's the thing: Companies expect to pay compensation for problems. Litigation, fines, and compensation costs are built into their business planning.

In 2021, four companies agreed to pay out $26 billion to settle claims relating to opioid abuse. This is what one attorney general had to say: "'This was a person-made crisis,' Josh Shapiro said at a press conference announcing the settlement. 'This epidemic was manufactured by an army of pharmaceutical executives.'" (Strickler, 2021).

The key takeaway here is that, in the grand scheme, pharmaceuticals are not produced with patients as their focus. No, the focus is profit. The pills you are prescribed are not necessarily the best treatment for your condition. They may just be the most profitable.

Clearly, there is a conflict of interest here, at least as far as doctor prescriptions are concerned. Doctors have to tell their patients if they have a financial interest or incentive to prescribe them with a particular medicine.

Symptom Treating

America spends more than twice as much on healthcare than other countries such as the UK, Canada, Australia, France, and New Zealand. (Tikkanen & Abrams, 2020). Out of the developed nations in the OECD, America has the greatest amount of chronic disease and obesity per capita. The country also has the highest number of hospitalizations and deaths from preventable causes.

The vast majority of drugs prescribed are only treating the symptoms. They rarely address the cause of the ailment. Treatments to fix the acid pains in your stomach are mostly just counteracting the acid and not actually dealing with whatever problem is the root cause. In all likelihood, it is your diet that is at fault.

A teacher friend of mine in the UK had chronic problems with acid reflux and stomach pains. After decades of being prescribed antacids and other symptom-treating drugs, he was referred to a GI clinic. The first question the consultant asked him was, "How much caffeine do you drink each day?"

There ended the consultation, and he was sent home to try a caffeine-free diet. The problem he had for decades disappeared. Just think how much had been spent on pointless treatments, not to mention the time taken up with GPs, the loss of workdays, and the cost to the community. Oh, and the years and years of pointless suffering.

Why?

Virtually every doctor he saw just wanted to treat the symptom. If the focus had been on the cause of his problems and finding out why he was suffering from these problems, then the problem would have been fixed immediately.

The irony is that his complaints concerned his digestive system. You know, where food goes. No other part of your body would be a more obvious place for your doctor to ask, "Hm. Maybe it's what they are eating?"

If doctors can't get the simple connection between diet and symptoms, what chance is there of finding relationships in more obscure parts of your body systems?

Furthermore, as this is the part of the body where nutrients are absorbed into the rest of the body, there is a good chance that the nutrients are not being absorbed as they should be, and therefore, messing up the rest of you.

What would a doctor do when he's driving his car and a red warning signal comes on? Maybe he thinks, "Oh, I better make sure that red light doesn't appear again." Then he cuts the wire to the warning light, the signal disappears, and the problem is fixed.

Except two weeks later, the car crashes into a ditch killing the doctor's entire family as water got into the brake fluid.

Sorry for the drama but, in effect, that is what our health system does to us: make the signal go away and make no effort to find out why we got that signal, resulting in the eventual failure of the machine that is you. To be clear, failure here means death, eventually.

We have a much more elaborate and sophisticated warning system than a car though—our nervous system. It lets us know, through pain and other signals, that something is wrong. Simply making the pain go away is worse than doing nothing. Now we are in a situation where there is still something fundamentally wrong, but it's not bothering us as much, so we don't worry about it. The root cause never gets fixed.

Like the doctor in his car, he stopped worrying as the red light was no longer flashing. The problem, though, was steadily getting worse.

The Problem of Specialism

Now, don't get me wrong. If I need brain surgery, I want the best brain specialist in the world to go digging in there. There is a reason why we have specialists in medicine. We need people who are highly trained in specific areas and techniques to do jobs that take years and years of training.

However, when you are sent to see a specialist, say a dermatologist, then their focus is likely to be on that body system. Other things that may be connected may not be considered. I say may, here, because some doctors now practice systems medicine. (Hyman, 2010).

With systems or functional medicine approaches, the doctor will run a series of tests on your cholesterol, vitamin and mineral levels, omega-3 fat levels, possible infections, allergies, and intolerances.

The aim of the tests is to identify what levels are too much, too little, or out of balance. The treatment that follows is to bring these back to good levels and restore balance. Normally, this involves making changes to the patient's diet and lifestyle—better nutrients, less ultra-processed foods, more exercise, and more sleep.

Often patients suffer from more than one ailment, and doctors look at each separately and treat each one separately, masking the underlying problems.

Yet, why wait until you are in a state of multiple problems and life-threatening conditions?

Let's go back to the car. You get your car serviced regularly. During that process, oil is topped up or replaced, clean water and antifreeze is added to the cooling system, brake fluids are topped up or replaced, battery acid levels are restored, window washer fluid is replenished, and so on. What the mechanic is doing is making sure that all the nutrients your car needs are at the correct levels.

Very few people wait until their engine seizes due to a lack of oil. We make sure that everything is tip-top so we don't have a huge bill when an unnecessary repair is needed or, for that matter, the car is written off.

Get your food right, and you won't need emergency balancing.

We are nearly finished with the gloom and doom part of the book. In the next chapter, we will stroll into the sunny uplands of how to maintain good health.

Overall, the reality is, simple doesn't cut it. Underlying causes need to be investigated and identified in order to achieve that wonderful state of being cured—actually cured.

Preventive Medicine

Just like looking after your car and getting it serviced regularly so that problems don't arise, preventive medicine focuses on making sure that your body and mind are being treated well and that you are getting the nutrients you need.

As much as 35% of cancers are due to poor diet, low activity, and obesity. ("Food as Preventative Medicine," n.d.). That is just one of the startling facts related to diseases in which diet is a huge factor.

The great thing is that by adopting a preventive approach to getting your diet right, you will vastly decrease your likelihood of developing a wide range of diseases. On top of that you will age slower and feel so much better, both mentally and physically.

In case you are getting anxious to find out what you need to do, here are the highlights:

- Get around 7–9 hours of sleep per night.
- Develop an exercise routine.
- Limit or even cut out red meat altogether.
- Reduce your intake of simple carbs.
- Keep to a balanced diet, including plenty of fruit and vegetables.
- Take vitamin and mineral supplements for any deficiencies you have.
- Avoid processed and ultra-processed foods, and have your diet focused on whole-grains and whole foods.
- Above all, keep your gut healthy.

That is basically it!

In the coming chapters, we will expand on this in more detail, looking at things like superfoods.

This book is about food and your health, but it would be remiss of me not to spell out what exercise you need (American Heart Association Editorial Staff, 2018):

- 150 minutes per week of moderate exercise spread throughout the week, or 75 minutes of vigorous aerobic exercise.
- Moderate to high-intensity muscle strengthening exercise with resistance bands or weights on two or more days per week.
- Reduce the amount of time you spend sitting down. If sitting is part of your job, then get a standing desk.
- Increase your activity to at least five hours per week as well as the intensity of your exercise.

Lifestyle change is not just something promoted in my books; clinicians have been given clear advice since 2007 that 75% of patient visits for a range of conditions should be focused on nutrition advice as a preventive medicine protocol. (Wallace, 2007).

The Body's Ability to Self-Heal

In your quest to seek the holy grail of good health, your knight in shining armor is your very own body and the cells it is made from. Unlike a car, your body can repair itself. To an extent, you are aware of this already. Every time you get a small cut or scratch, your body actually puts you back together again.

It does this through three main steps:

1. **Hemostasis.** Blood vessels contract to reduce bleeding, and platelets release fibrin proteins to clot the cut.
2. **Inflammation.** Yes, I know, inflammation is bad for you, but in this case, it is very good. The blood vessels expand, allowing more and more white blood cells to gather at the cut to fight any infectious invaders.
3. **Proliferation.** New skin cells grow over the wound.

As you can see, even in a simple case like this, your body has a shedfull of tools ready to be used as required. This—and other repair processes—have been built up over millions, even billions, of years of evolution. Since the earliest forms of life appeared, it was those with that little extra mutation tweak of self-repair that survived, passing their genes to the next generation.

The tiniest components of your body—cells—are very much like those early cells that developed repair mechanisms. They have the ability to repair damage to themselves and also to create replacements for cells that have died. A word of warning, though: Cerebral cortex neurons are not replaced when they die. Kill these cells off through things like too much alcohol, and they aren't coming back. Some of your cells, like heart muscle cells, have a slower rate of replacement as you get older. (Tom of AskaNaturalist.com, 2010).

The important takeaway from this is that you need to help your body in its self-healing mission. The help it needs—and it's hardly surprising—is good nutrition so that every part of you is getting the right nutrients in the amounts required. Nutrients are the essentials in the story of your body. Without them, the chain of events fails.

In addition to nutrition, your body's self-repair systems need you to exercise and, above all, get a decent night's sleep. Like the workers who come out to repair roads and railways when we are tucked up in bed, your body does most of its repair work when you are in the land of nod.

The End of the Beginning

Well, that's it for the first part of the book. In the rest of the book, we will be taking a profound look at the six pillars of health:

1. Food
2. Gut health
3. Immunity
4. Lifestyle
5. Stress
6. Sleep

Before we leave this section, what have we learned? Let's sum it up with what we started with.

Garbage in, garbage out. Unlike the sheep from Animal Farm, this mantra is not mindless. You have been introduced to the garbage—some of which you knew already, while some may have surprised you. Anyway, you now have a very good understanding of what constitutes the garbage you have been eating. Hopefully, you have taken the garbage out and, with a sense of mild guilt, left it for the raccoons.

Let's move on now and see what's coming in through the door to replace all that rubbish.

PART II
FOOD IS YOUR MEDICINE

> *One cannot think well, love well, sleep well, if one has not dined well.*
>
> –Virginia Wolfe

"ANNUAL INCOME TWENTY POUNDS, ANNUAL EXPENDITURE NINETEEN SIX, RESULT HAPPINESS. ANNUAL INCOME TWENTY POUNDS, ANNUAL EXPENDITURE TWENTY-POUND OUGHT SIX, RESULT MISERY."

— CHARLES DICKENS

CHAPTER 4:
THE BUILDING BLOCKS

This chapter is about the very basics of food and nutrition. I need to point out before we start that appendices A and B contain a lot more information related to this chapter.

The modern idea of using food as medicine started back in the 1980s with the AIDs epidemic. Nutrition programs were conceived that helped with the management of the disease. This developed into the Food Is Medicine Coalition (FIMC). ("Food Is Medicine Coalition," n.d.). The good thing about this organization is that their advice is evidence-based.

Around 80% of all chronic diseases and premature deaths are preventable simply by focusing on good nutrition, smoking cessation, and exercise. (Katch, 2017).

Food as Medicine

We have examined the negative effects of a lot of foodstuffs and also covered aspects of good nutrition. Chapter five is where we will look at how a healthy diet can keep diseases at bay. However, many studies have clearly indicated the link between diet and disease, especially the big killers like heart disease, stroke, type 2 diabetes, and cancer. (Micha et al., 2017).

Eating too much processed food, red meat, sugary drinks, and salt are the villains, and fruits, vegetables, nuts, seeds, whole-grains, polyunsaturated fats, and omega-3 fatty acids (mainly from seafood) are the good guys.

Food is a hot topic. It seems like every month there is a new diet on the block, and it can be bewildering for anyone to decide just what they should do beyond the basics of don't eat the rubbish mentioned above and do eat more of the good stuff, but which of the many diets out there are good and which are passing fads?

The only sure tool of discrimination is to ensure that the diet is evidence-based, and by that, I don't mean the website or book is full of references to what the author regards as evidence, but evidence that is based on peer-reviewed scientific research. In other words, data that is sourced from the scientific method where the main job of the scientist with a hypothesis is to test how it can be wrong, exhaustively. Their fellow scientists then try to prove it wrong as well. This is why it can take a long time from stating a hypothesis to coming out with concrete conclusions. (Lumen Learning, n.d.).

For some diets, like the Keto, Portfolio, and DASH diets, good evidence backs up their claims. Some diets combine other diets, like the MIND diet, which draws from the DASH and Mediterranean diets and may be good at preventing Alzheimer's. The MIND diet revolves more around berries and leafy green vegetables.

In one study, the diet indicated it could prevent cognitive aging in women by two and a half years. (Higuera, 2017).

On the other hand, there is no conclusive evidence that a gluten-free diet is of benefit to the population at large.

One thing to remember is that nutrition-based medicine complements modern medicine. It is by no means a replacement. It acts more as a preventive measure.

When you do develop a disease, nutrition can also help ameliorate or cure the condition. Sometimes, a change in diet is all you need. However, there are many ailments that require modern cures. You can't eat your way out of COVID-19. Having a good healthy body supported by quality nutrition will lessen your risk of severe results, though.

The Data Speaks

One in nine people in the world are malnourished. These people just can't get enough food, never mind the right foods. In the developed world, well, the world is our oyster; we can eat whatever we want and as much as we want. Our problem is not a lack of food but too much food and too much choice.

Throughout the book, so far, we have highlighted the statistics that show how much of a difference good nutrition can deliver. The data is very significant.

Over the decades, nutrition scientists have managed to separate out the multitude of components that make up our food and to find out exactly what they do to us, good and bad.

For example, it is from that research we can confidently say you need zinc for the following:

> *Formation of enzymes, new cells and proteins, your immune system, taste, smell, wound healing, and for releasing vitamin A from the liver. Recommended daily amount (RDA) is 11 mg. Safe upper limit (UL) is 40 mg. Vegetarians need to supplement.*

That is an extract from appendix B. Most people read books and ignore the appendices. However, the appendices go into much more detail, as succinctly as possible.

The Food Matrix

I love impressive, science names like matrix. But let's not get too technical. As mentioned above and in appendix B, there are required amounts of a range of nutrients that your body needs to function in all of its parts. The danger of that knowledge is to assume that you can get away with just swallowing capsule or pill supplements. Come on, hands up; who was thinking that?

Our bodies are not designed to consume micronutrients like an amoeba. We are engineered to eat foods. The reason why just gulping pills is a bad idea is because there is a complex interplay between nutrients and our digestive systems (including your gut bacteria) taking place. This is the matrix.

Taking supplements or fortified foods can result in poor absorption of a nutrient, overdosing on nutrients that are toxic, and missing out on key interactions with other nutrients.

THE BUILDING BLOCKS

We mentioned iron earlier, but it is worth remembering that the body cannot absorb iron on its own and too much can be toxic, damaging to the gut, and give us constipation and nausea.

To be absorbed, iron has to be part of protein molecules. With the iron bound in this way, it cannot damage your gut. Here's another element from the matrix: Consuming iron-rich foods along with foods rich in vitamin C will allow you to absorb the iron better. Consuming iron foods along with a lot of dietary fiber can significantly lower the absorption rate. Our digestive system is complex because it deals with complex foods. That is no accident. Again, do I have to say, "millions of years of evolution?"

From this matrix, we develop dietary patterns; in other words, foods that should be combined to promote good health. Although the advice in the appendices indicates what foods have which nutrients, it is not enough to consider eating individual foods. That's not a diet; it's Russian roulette with your stomach.

Food as Information

Like those episodes in science fiction where the hero gives data to a mad robot that it cannot compute and blows up, food is also data. Give your body the wrong data, and it malfunctions. Give it the right data, and it operates like a well-oiled machine.

Let's look at one example: For our immune system to work correctly, the information required must contain vitamins A, B6, C, E, riboflavin, and the minerals: folic acid, magnesium, selenium, and zinc. These are the instructions that our cells take in to output things like antibodies. The various outputs may contain these micronutrients, and some of the micronutrients are needed for the process that creates the output to function.

Our cells are remarkably complex, with power sources that need fuel, factories that need raw materials, transport systems for receiving and delivering, and a control system to make sure everything happens in the right sequence and at the right time.

They also have a fence with gates in it (the cell membrane) that has to be maintained. The gates that let stuff in and out need things like sodium in order to function.

Another thing to consider is that one piece of information can end up with different meanings depending on which cells are using it. As an example, we could go with any mineral or vitamin, but let's choose selenium. It is needed for the following:

- Building certain enzymes and proteins needed for DNA
- Protecting against cell damage
- Fighting infections
- Allowing certain processes in reproduction
- Metabolizing thyroid hormones

Those are just its day jobs. As a powerful antioxidant, it helps to reduce the risk of cancers, heart disease, and mental decline.

We mostly think of food as a source of energy for building materials for the body, but there is so much more to food than that. This information perspective helps us to understand that processes in our body will cease to function properly if the right information doesn't arrive at the right time.

Disease and Food

At one time, diseases like cancers, type 2 diabetes, stroke, heart disease, and even obesity were thought to be caused by gene mutations. That's why you are often asked if there is a history of a condition in your family.

Now, while genes are of major importance, it is also now recognized that disease arises as a result of a complex interplay between genes and the environment. The most significant part of our environment is what we eat.

Genes—good and bad—can be turned on or off. Turning them on is known as gene expression. All sorts of environmental factors, such as tobacco smoke, can cause latent genes to express, resulting in things like cancer.

Our food has that power too. The science of nutrigenomics studies the link between nutrients in our food and the additions or subtractions that are made to chemical marks on our DNA, and the switching on or off of genes. (Kirkpatrick, 2018).

We are now looking closely at how combinations of specific nutrients affect the various functions of the body.

Functional Medicine

Practitioners of functional medicine approach disease from the view that nutrition plays a major role in a variety of systems in the body and that these systems interact with each other. They also have the view that disease is very often preceded by an overall decline in the general health of the patient.

With this in mind, they are keen to identify patients in this declining phase so that they can intervene with good nutritional adjustments to prevent the milder symptoms from developing into a full-blown disease.

A key principle is that one disease might be the result of several causes as well as one problem being the underlying cause for several diseases. Identifying these nutrient causes is the path to ensuring that diseases don't develop.

Nutrition 101

Why Don't We Eat a Healthy Diet

There are two main reasons why we don't eat a healthy diet even though we know we should. The first reason is that we only think about the bad foods.

Over the years, authorities have constantly been telling us what foods are bad. Things like carbs, red meat, and fats. If you were to ask people what constituted a good diet, they might reply with "five fruits and vegetables a day."

So the focus has mainly been on bad rather than good eating habits.

The other problem is that people are just not changing their habits despite knowing what they should do. Since 1991, consumption of fruit and vegetables in America hasn't increased.

So, how do you change? The only sure way is to develop habits. You need to plan your meals rather than leaving things to the last minute. Plan a week in advance so that you have the ingredients available each day.

Follow these 10 steps:

1. **Eat a wide variety of foods.** So, it's not just a case of eating fruit, vegetables, whole-grains, meat, legumes, fish, nuts, seeds, and seafood. You need to vary your diet within these categories. If you are just eating the same whole-grains or the same legumes, then you will find yourself missing out on nutrients that are found in other varieties.

2. **Don't just stick to five-a-day for fruits and vegetables.** The recommendation from the USDA Center for Nutrition Policy is for between 5–13 per day. Five is the bare minimum. Plants have a chemical arsenal known as phytochemicals that protect them from fungi, bacteria, viruses, insects, and animals. ("Phytochemical," n.d.). The great thing is that when we eat plants, these chemicals become our phytonutrients, and they help us fight a whole range of diseases. To get a good range of these nutrients, you need to eat a range of colors—green, yellow-orange, blue-purple, red, and white. For example, tomatoes, especially cooked tomatoes, give us lycopene, and carrots contain carotenoids. Fruit and vegetables are also good for our gut bacteria and provide us with fiber.

3. **Eat whole grains.** This provides us with fiber and a range of nutrients. Processed grains can lose up to 95% of specific nutrients.

4. **Keep fats in your diet.** Your body needs omega-6 and omega-3 fatty acids to function. Omega-6, we get through animal fats and corn oil. They are needed for our immune system. Our health as a nation is poor as a result of

inflammation caused by having too much omega-6 in our diet and not enough omega-3. We need inflammation, as it is a part of our immune system's defense mechanisms. The important thing here is to have a balance between the two. A low amount of omega-3 compared to omega-6 can lead to inflammation, diabetes, atherosclerosis, rheumatoid arthritis, and heart failure. In the west, the ratio of omega-6 to omega-3 in our diets is about 16:1. We evolved to have a ratio of 1:1. It is recommended that you should have a ratio of 2:1. (Ajmera, 2009).

5. **Drink water.** Your body is composed mainly of water. If you don't keep yourself topped up, then your health will suffer. Men should drink about 3 liters of water per day, and women should consume 2.2 liters. Around 20% of your water should come from what you eat—fruits, vegetables, and so on.

6. **Drink green tea.** It contains very powerful antioxidants and, according to various studies, it may benefit you by reducing cancer risk, boosting your brain function, increasing fat-burning, controlling your blood sugar, and reducing your risk of heart disease. If you are iron deficient, then leave any tea drinking to when you are not eating, as the tannins in teas reduce iron absorption. (Lewin, 2023).

7. **Don't overeat.** For a long time now, we have known that calorie restriction is a good way to slow down aging. Sticking to the foods recommended in this book will help with that. Use smaller plates to eat from, as this will prevent you from eating too much by "cleaning your plate."

Intermittent fasting, where you have a period of 16 hours or more every day when you don't eat, is a very effective way of controlling calorie intake too.

8. **Don't eat hydrogenated or trans fats.** These are very far from natural, as it involves an industrial process to convert normal vegetable oils into fats. Unfortunately, these trans fats are treated by the body as ordinary fats, but they don't function the same. Always check food labels for trans fats. Of course, if you don't eat processed foods, then you won't have anything to worry about.

9. **Don't eat artificial sweeteners like corn syrup.** Too much of these can lead to obesity and type 2 diabetes. Ordinary sucrose, like table sugar, triggers the body to produce a hormone called leptin that makes you feel full. Corn syrup and other sweeteners don't.

10. **Cut down or even eliminate processed foods.** These are normally high in sugars, salt, and additives while being low in essential nutrients.

The Healthy Diet

We started this chapter with a quote from jolly old Mr. Micawber in Charles Dickens' *David Copperfield*. While he was speaking about income, the same reasoning applies to calorie intake—in reverse. We need around 2,000 calories a day to function. Taking in more than that will lead to an increase in the storage of calories in our bodies—in fat cells.

Fat cells have many functions, but the main function is to store energy for a rainy day for times of starvation. In the west, we don't really have periods of starvation, so eating more calories than we need on a regular basis just results in our fat cells storing more and more fats.

If you are overweight, then to lose that extra weight, you need to either burn more calories through exercise or eat less than your required daily amount. In actual fact, they are the same thing. Exercise burns calories because you are using more than you are taking in. If, after exercise, you satisfy your hunger with a "well-deserved" blowout, then you are defeating the weight-loss point of the exercise.

But whatever diet you are following, it must have the following elements:

- **Calorie control.** Adjust your calorie intake depending on whether you wish to gain or lose weight.
- **Variety.** Nutrients are not conveniently packaged in a single food. To get the correct levels of nutrients your body needs, you must eat as wide a variety of foods as you can.
- **Moderation.** Avoid extremes. Don't eat too much of one thing or too little of another.
- **Adequacy.** A good diet must have enough nutrients, fiber, and calories to sustain a healthy body.
- **Balance.** Make sure you get the appropriate amount of each nutrient.

Being a Food Sleuth

Fortunately, you don't need to be a Marlowe or Poirot to find out what is in the food you are buying. There are no hidden secrets to be unearthed by clever detective work. It is all there on the label.

THE BUILDING BLOCKS

Research shows that almost two-thirds of Americans read food labels. (Coast Packing Company, 2016). For most, though, it will be the main headlines they are looking for, calories, salt, sugar, and fats. There is, however, much more that you need to know to get the best out of each label.

Before we look at this though, it's worthwhile to note that there is vital information that is not legally required on labels. These are the amounts of the following:

- Potassium
- Essential minerals and vitamins (only a, c, calcium, and iron are legally required)
- Sugar alcohol
- Soluble fiber
- Other carbohydrates
- Calories from saturated fats
- Polyunsaturated fats
- Monounsaturated fats.
- Vitamin a present as beta-carotene
- Genetically modified organisms

So, there is a lot hidden that is really worth knowing. The above list is optional. Manufacturers don't need to include them. Of course, they may include the good stuff like vitamins and minerals while leaving out the bad news.

Be careful to note that the figures quoted on the label are per serving size too.

When reading the label, here are the things to be aware of:

> ➤ The daily percentage value is based on an intake of 2,000 calories.
>   - 5% of a daily value is low.
>   - 20% of a daily value is high.
> ➤ An information panel at the bottom indicates the maximum amount of fat, cholesterol, and sodium that should be in your daily diet. Remember, these are maximums and not targets!
> ➤ Organic means that 95% of the ingredients come from natural sources. The other 5% can be various additives or other ingredients.

The USA and the EU are broadly similar in their food labeling requirements. The main difference is that in the US, additives are indicated by their common names whereas in the EU, they are listed as three- or four-digit E numbers.

However, when it comes to what additives are allowed, the EU is much stricter. Additives are only allowed if they have been proved to be unharmful. Consequently, there are many additives of a petrochemical nature in American foods that are banned in the EU. ("EU versus US," 2018).

Health and Qualified Health Claims

Often, on the packaging, you will see claims such as "reduces heart disease" and "supportive but no conclusive research shows..." The first of these is a full-on health claim that has been proven by scientific research. Notice, though, that it doesn't claim to cure the disease. The second example is a qualified health claim. In this case, there are research indications that the food may be beneficial for some aspect of health. However, more research is needed before the evidence becomes conclusive.

A third class of health claim is the structure or function claim, where the manufacturer is allowed to state that the food may boost your immune system, for example. These must also include a disclaimer that the FDA hasn't evaluated the claim.

Allergies

There are eight ingredients that must appear on the food label, if it contains them. These are peanuts, wheat, soy, eggs, milk, tree nuts, fish, and shellfish. In the EU, there are 14 allergens that must be listed.

Remember, though, that individuals can be allergic to just about anything. In my circle of friends and family, there are allergies to oats, ginger, cinnamon, chicken, and a range of berries and fruits.

If you think you may have an allergy, then you need to get tested so you can eliminate it from your diet.

Balancing Your Meals

You are bombarded by the media, by friends and family, and in emails with exhortations to eat this, avoid that, and stick to the latest fad diet daily. It is no wonder that we don't know what we should or shouldn't be doing.

The problem is that catchy headline diets tend to make you focus on one aspect of your diet, and you lose the width that is necessary for a balanced diet.

Let's start with the nutrients your body needs. There are six of these:

1. Proteins
2. Carbohydrates
3. Lipids (fats)
4. Vitamins
5. Minerals
6. Water

A healthy, balanced diet must include all of these. In our foods, many of these are combined. For example, lipids often contain fat-soluble vitamins. What you eat to get these is even simpler. There are three core food groups. Your diet should be composed of the following:

> **25% protein.** This is needed for growth and repair. This is where we come back to something I mentioned earlier: Keep it varied. Don't get into the habit of eating one source of protein. Note that dairy products are included here, and you need to think of them as a subgroup due to their calcium content.

> **50% fruit and vegetables** (including nuts, seeds, and herbs). This is your healthy metabolism source. They are loaded with vitamins and minerals. Many of these are powerful antioxidants. They are also sources of fiber, which helps your digestive system and helps you with weight control as they give a feeling of fullness.

> **25% carbohydrates.** These are the gas in your car. They are your primary source of energy. Stick to whole-grain carbohy-

drates, as they are rich in fiber and vitamin B. The more active you are, then the more carbohydrates you will need.

So, that's your diet plan. Stick to those portions and ensure variety, and your diet will be balanced.

Remember that every meal that you eat doesn't have to be balanced, so long as, over the course of a few days, you are getting enough of each food group. For example, If you eat an apple, you don't have to start thinking, "I must have a bit of salmon with that on whole-grain toast."

We have covered the dangers of processed foods and especially ultra-processed foods. However, if you have a cake, chocolate, or even chips once in a while, then it is not going to cause havoc to your system. The problem is that with many of these foods, they are habit-forming or even addictive.

The Functions of Foods

Taking forward the brief information in the previous section, let's dive a little deeper into what these foods do to you.

Nutrients and Genes

In fact, let's plumb the depths to begin with. Genes are the most basic elements of you. They decide everything from hair color to causing diseases. However, it is factors in our environment that cause the disease-causing genes to switch on or be expressed.

Nutrigenomics is a relatively new science that is focused on how nutrients interact with our genes. The possible future outcome of this science is that people may end up having individualized diets depending on their genetic profile and disease risks. (Nutrigenomics, 2018). One study comparing the effect of a rye-based diet with a wheat-based alternative showed that the risk of diabetes due to gene expression was lowered in the rye diet.

Fruits and Vegetables

Fruits and vegetables are a rich source of vitamins and minerals, as well as fiber and phytonutrients. Fiber slows down carbohydrate absorption and helps us feel full. The defensive phytonutrients contained in plants help to reduce inflammation. The role of vitamins and minerals is complex, and often they interact with each other. They play a vital role in most metabolic processes. Appendix B has a rundown on the various functions of each mineral and vitamin.

Remember to eat the rainbow! Plants of different colors have different phytonutrients that help our bodies.

Aside from the variety of colors, you should be aiming to eat at least five portions of fruit and vegetables per day. Ideally, you should aim for as many as 13.

Whole-Grains

When we hear about whole grains, we usually think of three benefits: fiber, fiber, and fiber.

Their role in your health is so much more than that. In fact, there are seven very clear benefits:

1. Manufacturing of neurotransmitters such as serotonin
2. Improves the functioning of the digestive system

3. Reducing cholesterol
4. Removing toxins from your body
5. Appetite control due to making you feel full
6. Encouraging healthy bacteria, which assist digestion
7. Regulates blood sugar due to slowing down the digestion of carbohydrates

To improve your health, look out for "whole grain" on the ingredients list, and cut down on the amount of refined grains you eat.

Proteins

In most people's heads, protein is associated with muscle. We often assume that if we aren't into bodybuilding, then we don't really need a lot of protein. So, let's look at the eight functions proteins are needed for.

1. Building muscle, as expected
2. Strengthening connective tissue, which is needed in bone, skin, and cartilage
3. Wound healing
4. Assisting thyroid and adrenal function
5. Helping you feel full
6. Detoxification, as the liver binds waste molecules to proteins so that they can be removed from your body
7. Hormone and enzyme production, since enzymes are predominantly composed of proteins, and hormones are made of proteins and amino acids. (Some enzymes play vital roles in digesting food)
8. Controlling insulin and blood sugar balance

The protein we eat is broken down into amino acids through digestion. In our cells, the amino acids are reassembled into the proteins we need. To ensure you have all the amino acids required, it is important to keep your protein sources as varied as possible. Vegan diets need to source proteins from grains, legumes, nuts, and seeds. A lack of variety can lead to mood disorders, poor tissue repair, and cognitive dysfunction. (Giampapa, 2019).

Fats and Oils

The black sheep of the family, or so they are perceived. The word fat is often used as a derogatory term, so it is little wonder why we mostly see fats as bad. But they are necessary and not in the pejorative view of a "necessary evil." There are no less than 10 major functions for fats and oils:

1. Needed for the production of hormones
2. Improving gut health
3. Lubrication of skin and mucous membranes
4. Healthy joints
5. Ingestion of fat-soluble vitamins (A, D, E, and K)
6. Insulating our organs
7. Helping our immune system
8. Better use of glucose
9. Regulation of inflammation
10. Healthy and functional cell membranes

Reduce the amount of saturated fats and try to get the bulk of your necessary fats from fish and plants.

Portion Size

You might not be aware, but over the decades, what we regard as a portion has changed in size. There are no prizes for guessing that they have increased. Take a simple coffee, for example. Back in the day, coffee with whole milk and sugar was about eight ounces and had a slimline 45 calories. Flash-forward to today's sophisticated mocha with syrup and steamed whole milk, and not only has the portion doubled to 16 ounces, but the calorie content has ballooned to 350 calories, nearly eight times as much.

As a nation and as individuals, we have gradually gotten used to food being available and relatively cheap. Overtime, we have conditioned ourselves to eat more. If you bought a chocolate chip cookie today, you would be very disappointed if you discovered it was from 30 years ago and was only a fifth of a modern one.

So, not only do we have to rethink what we are eating but also how much.

To help you judge what a correct portion size is, follow this ready reckoner.

Food	Portion Size Equivalent
3 ounces of fish	Smartphone
3 ounces of meat and poultry	Deck of cards
1 ounce of cheese	2 dice
2 tablespoons of peanut butter	Ping-Pong ball

LET FOOD BE YOUR MEDICINE

Seeds and nuts	1 large egg
Rice, mashed potatoes, pasta, and beans	Tennis ball
Cereal	1 closed fist
Butter or oil	Thumb down to the first joint
Leafy greens	Baseball
Fruit and vegetables	Light bulb
Dried fruit	Golf ball

One of my Scottish friends told me that his father often said, "Yir eyes are bigger than yir belly" when he had filled his plate with way more than he could eat. The problem now is that, psychologically, our bellies have evolved to match our eyes. We see a heaped plateful of food, and we keep going until there is nothing left.

Control that by doing the following:

- ➢ Stick to the recommended portion sizes above when making up your plate.
- ➢ No going back for seconds or thirds!
- ➢ No overeating in restaurants simply to clear your plate. Get the rest bagged to go.
- ➢ Use a smaller plate.
- ➢ Don't eat until you are stuffed.
- ➢ Increase the fiber in your diet, as this will make you feel full.

Beverages

We often forget that we get a lot of our calories and nutrients through what we drink. A gram of alcohol has 7 calories, which is nearly as much as fat at 9 calories per gram. (NHS, n.d.). Now you know where beer bellies come from.

Water is a very safe beverage in terms of nutrition and health. It is essential. Yet, with most meals, we tend to drink something else.

Sugary drinks are the worst culprit. A regular 16-ounce drink of mocha, soda, or an energy drink will have more than 50 g of sugar. That's almost 200 calories.

Fruit drinks are often sweetened. It is best to make sure that you are drinking 100% unsweetened fruit juice.

In the next chapter, we will expand on our investigation into nutrients by taking a closer look at the different classes and what they do.

> EAT BREAKFAST LIKE A KING, LUNCH LIKE A PRINCE, AND DINNER LIKE A PAUPER.
>
> — ADELE DAVIS

CHAPTER 5:
STEPPING UP YOUR NUTRITION GAME

In the last chapter, we were mainly concerned with the macronutrients like carbohydrates, proteins, and lipids. In a way, these are the things we see on our plates. Contained within those macronutrients are the micronutrients, which are the things we can't see and only know about due to modern science.

This is an advantage that we have over more ancient humans. At the beginning of the 20th century, the only nutrients known were proteins, carbohydrates, and fats.

During the first half of the century, all the vitamins we know now were discovered. As the years have progressed, we have come to understand more and more of what these essential components do in the various systems and processes of the body. (Tweed, 2021).

Vitamins and Minerals

We have talked a lot about these throughout the book and will continue to do so due to their fundamental role in maintaining a healthy body, but just what do they do?

Before we get to that, the fundamental difference between minerals and vitamins is that the former are simple inorganic elements from the periodic table, found in soil and water, and are passed to us by plants or by animals that eat plants. They are the simplest components of ordinary matter.

Vitamins, on the other hand, are complex organic molecules that are made within living creatures. In fact, our bodies are capable of making vitamins D and K. When we expose our skin to sunlight our bodies produce vitamin D. Vitamin K2 is made in our gut by the good bacteria that live there. There is only one form of Vitamin K1, and it is produced by plants. K2 has 12 different forms only one of which is made from vitamin K1. The other 11 forms are either made in our gut or are ingested from animals that have made them in their gut. (Busch, 2018).

All the rest of the vitamins and minerals we need are in our food, well, if we are eating the right foods. In appendix B, you will find all the information you need on what each vitamin and mineral does and how much we need.

Multivitamins?

If you have a properly balanced diet, then you will get all the vitamins that your body needs. However, there are occasions when these need to be supplemented. If, for example, you are diagnosed with a specific deficiency, or you live in a part of the world where food varieties are limited, you may need to purchase vitamins outside those you get from your diet.

Over 90% of Americans do not ingest enough vitamin C or D. ("Should I Take A Daily Multivitamin," 2021). For the vast majority, this could be rectified by a change to a more healthy diet.

The older you get, the more difficult it becomes to absorb vitamin B12 from food. If you are over the age of 50, then you should be taking vitamin B12 supplements.

Pregnant women also need to take 600 mcg of folic acid per day to reduce the risk of anencephaly or spina bifida.

Those who suffer from low bone density need to take supplemental calcium and vitamin D3.

In addition to these, there are malabsorption conditions and medicines that reduce the amount of vitamins getting into our blood that require supplementation.

Diseases Related to Vitamin and Mineral Deficiency

A lack of vitamin C causes scurvy. Americans often refer to the British as Limeys due to the practice adopted in the British navy of eating citrus fruits to ward off scurvy.

Blindness can be caused by a lack of vitamin A and is still a problem in poorer countries.

Vitamin D is essential to healthy bones. In early life, a lack of the vitamin D can lead to rickets and, in later life, to osteopenia and osteoporosis. Since the 1930s, American milk has been fortified with vitamin D to reduce the problems associated with the lack of this essential nutrient.

The foxhole brother of vitamin D is calcium. Without adequate amounts of calcium, we can't develop or maintain healthy bones and teeth, and both are needed.

Interactions

Well, we have just seen that vitamin D is needed to extract calcium from our foods, but too much will result in magnesium deficiencies. Likewise, we also need vitamin C to absorb iron, but it has a detrimental effect on copper absorption. Too much vitamin A, though, and our ability to absorb vitamin K decreases and can decrease vitamin D absorption by 30%, but vitamin A needs zinc to be absorbed itself. So, all in all, it's a sophisticated world out there. (HealthAid, 2021).

Even medium levels of vitamin E can drastically reduce vitamin D absorption, and too much folic acid can cause symptoms of vitamin B12 deficiency.

These are just some of the interplays. Some of them are good and others are bad. The important thing to remember is that a balanced diet ensures that you get your vitamins and minerals in amounts that are beneficial.

Water-Soluble Vitamins

These are the easiest vitamins for our bodies to deal with. When you eat food containing vitamin C or the range of B vitamins, they enter the bloodstream easily. At the same time, your kidneys are getting rid of excess water-soluble vitamins to prevent harmful buildups of these.

These vitamins need to be topped up every few days, though some can last in your body for a long time. Vitamin B12, for example, can be stored in the liver for years.

There are four main functions of these vitamins:

1. B vitamins help to form coenzymes that assist enzymes in releasing energy from food.
2. Five of the B vitamins—riboflavin, thiamin, niacin, biotin, and pantothenic acid—are needed for energy production.
3. Vitamins B6 and B12 are needed, along with iron, to metabolize amino acids, assisting in the building of proteins.
4. Collagen is needed in our bodies as a base for teeth and bones. It is also needed to support blood vessel walls and knit together wounds. Vitamin C is a vital component in making collagen.

Fat-Soluble Vitamins

The process of absorbing these vitamins is rather more complicated than for their water-soluble siblings. Most of the work is done in the small intestine, where bile from the liver helps to break down fats. The vitamins released then pass through the wall of the small intestine into lymph vessels, where they are coupled with a protein, overwhelmingly, before entering the bloodstream.

Vitamins that aren't absorbed on the voyage through the body are absorbed by the liver or fat cells. Those in the liver can be released back into the bloodstream as required by the body.

They don't have to be consumed as often as water-soluble vitamins due to this storage effect. The fat-soluble vitamins are A, D, E, and K.

They mainly work to keep your nervous system, skin, eyes, lungs, and GI tract healthy, but they also do the following:

1. To build bones, A, D, and K are required.
2. Vitamin A is needed to maintain good vision.
3. Without vitamin E, your body finds the absorption and storage of vitamin A difficult. They support each other.
4. Vitamin E is also an antioxidant, protecting your body from disease-causing free radicals.

Due to long-term storage of these vitamins in the liver, taking too many supplements over a prolonged period can lead to toxic levels of these vitamins.

Once again, a balanced diet ensures that you get these in the correct quantities.

Major Minerals

There are seven major minerals that your body needs: sodium, chloride, potassium, calcium, phosphorus, magnesium, and sulfur. (NIH, 2018). They are needed in fairly large quantities and play important roles. Calcium alone can account for up to 1.2 kg of body mass.

The first three—sodium, chloride, and potassium—are vital for maintaining the balance of water in your body.

The following three—calcium, phosphorus, and magnesium—are needed for healthy bones. Phosphorus is also a key element in cell membranes.

The final mineral—sulfur—is required for stabilizing protein structures, especially in nails, hair, and skin.

Too much salt or sodium can result in the excretion of calcium, as calcium binds to sodium. Magnesium absorption is hindered by too much phosphorus as well.

Trace Minerals

Unlike the major minerals, trace minerals exist in our bodies in very small quantities but are nevertheless essential to the functioning of our body systems. They are: "chromium, copper, fluoride, iodine, iron, manganese, molybdenum, selenium, and zinc." (Lehman, 2021).

Iron gives the red color to our blood and is a key element in hemoglobin, which transports oxygen around the body. Fluoride, of course, is needed for healthy teeth and bones.

Related to iron is copper, as it is needed for an enzyme that helps with the metabolism of iron. In addition, it is a key element in a range of other enzymes.

Zinc is intimately involved in the immune system and helps your blood to clot.

In addition, if you don't have enough iodine, then hormones produced by the thyroid gland will diminish, leading to weight gain and lethargy. This is exacerbated if you don't have enough selenium.

The difference between too little of some of these trace minerals and too much is not wide. As a result, you need to be cautious when taking supplements so that you are not causing problems by having too much. As we require them in small amounts, we can get all we need through a balanced diet.

Antioxidants

Free radicals! No, it's not a call to liberate Bolivian revolutionaries. They are, in fact, charged particles roaming around our bodies, looking to cause damage by sucking electrons off other molecules they meet on the way.

Unfortunately, when they do that, this can cause changes in the behavior of the molecule. In our bodies, the molecule most often identified with free radical damage is DNA. They also damage cell membranes and other functional components of cells. It's generally not a good idea to let something mess with the blueprint of you.

Antioxidants work by giving their own electrons to neutralize the free radicals. (Harvard Health Publishing, 2019). Think of them as the secret service agent taking a bullet for the president.

Now, our highly evolved immune system produces its own antioxidants to fight this threat. However, increasing the amount of antioxidants in your diet will dramatically affect the prevalence of these health-threatening chemicals.

Simple things like cooked tomatoes provide lycopene, quercetin in apples and onions, catechins in green tea, and flavonoids such as those found in blueberries are excellent antioxidants. So, too, are vitamins C, E, and selenium.

Nutrient Deficiencies

Deficiencies of particular nutrients are usually due to a poor diet. Either you are not eating the right things and are missing out on some key nutrients, or you are eating the wrong things, which are preventing the absorption of nutrients.

Remember that having too much of one nutrient may affect the levels of another critical nutrient.

Having that broad, balanced diet is a major step in ensuring you don't have deficiencies.

When you do have deficiencies, though, the signs can be quite varied.

Let's start with a common one. A lack of vitamin B12 can reveal itself as anemia—swollen tongue, weakness, fatigue, cognitive problems, memory loss, balance problems, and numbness or tingling in your hands and feet.

Remember that as we go through these symptoms, they are indicators of a deficiency, but they may be caused by something else. It's always best to seek medical advice for severe symptoms.

Vegetarians, and especially vegans, are more at risk, as plants don't make B12. If you are practicing these types of diets, then you need to make sure you are eating grains fortified with B12 or taking supplements. Don't worry about those supplements being sourced from animals, though. B12 is made in the gut by bacteria, and supplements simply use bacterial cultures to produce B12. (McFarland, 2020).

Anemia, of course, is also caused by iron deficiency, and, like B12, the first signs are often fatigue. Indeed, a deficiency in vitamin D can also signal its lack through fatigue as well. My colon cancer was diagnosed after a colonoscopy because my internist discovered I was anemic. His search for a reason why I was anemic saved my life.

Fatigue can also be caused by a lack of vitamin C and most of the other B vitamins. This is why it is important to seek a diagnosis from a doctor.

You need to identify what is actually causing the symptom. Remember that you should try to find doctors that practice functional medicine.

A decrease in vitamins A, B, C, and D can be manifested in dry skin and hair. Depression may result from a deficiency in B vitamins 1, 3, 6, 9, and our old friend 12. However, it can also be caused by low vitamin C or D levels. Again, another reminder, these are *possible* causes, not *definite* causes.

If you find that you bruise easily or cuts don't heal quickly, then it could be due to a deficiency in vitamins C or K. Poor wound healing can also be caused by a lack of vitamins A, B, and D.

Keep getting the sniffles? Seem to catch every cold going? Then your immune system might be crying out for vitamins A, C, and D. If it is A that is low, then you have a much greater risk of diarrhea, malaria, measles, chronic ear infections, and respiratory diseases.

A friend of mine managed to get a hairline fracture in his right humerus. (Don't ask why!) After a bone scan, it turned out he had osteopenia. He was immediately put on calcium and vitamin D3. However, low bone density can also be caused by low levels of vitamins A, B6, B9, B12, C, and K.

If your friends are solicitously informing you that you look pale or you have noticed darker spots losing their pigmentation, then you could be lacking vitamin B6, B9, B12, C, or D.

Let's finish by looking at a short list of symptoms that are often caused, but not exclusively, by nutrient deficiencies:

- ➢ Fatigue or weakness
- ➢ Muscle cramps or twitches
- ➢ Numbness or tingling
- ➢ Not being able to think clearly

To get a fuller picture, look at the information collated in appendix B.

When to Eat

Is there a best time to eat? Well, like little wind-up dolls, we run on clockwork or, to give them the scientific veneer, circadian rhythms.

I've mentioned evolution a lot throughout the text, and here I go again. We evolved to sleep at night and be active during the day. A nexus of 20,000 neurons in the brain is our master clock. It has been developed by millions of years of evolution. Our digestive system fits into the rhythm. We are designed to eat during daylight hours. Eating late at night, before sleep, is outside this natural time frame. It can increase the risk of cancer, diabetes, and heart disease. (NIH, 2023).

At night, when we are asleep, our resistance to insulin peaks. As a result, late-night snacking or midnight feasts result in most of the calories being converted to fat.

This chapter started with a quote from Adlel Davis' book, *Let's Eat Right to Keep Fit*. (Davis, 1954). Eating most of your food in the morning means that you are giving your body the energy it needs for its daily activities. Not only that but as a result of only eating lightly in the evening, you avoid the risk of fat building up as you sleep.

Allied to the time of day is the need for regularity. Just like needing a settled sleep cycle, we also thrive better when our eating times occur at the same times each day and don't skip about.

The best eating pattern involves the following:

- ➢ Eat most calories earlier in the day.
- ➢ Don't eat too close to bedtime.
- ➢ Have at least 12 hours per day, including sleeping, when you are not eating.
- ➢ Don't eat as soon as you rise.

This last point seems to contradict the "Eat breakfast like a king" mantra. However, it is for exactly the same reason as not eating late at night. During sleep, melatonin is released, reducing insulin release, which, in turn, reduces the uptake of glucose by cells.

When you get up in the morning, it takes time for the melatonin to subside to its normal levels. Therefore, you should leave breakfast after the feeling of drowsiness wears off.

Currently, there are variations in eating times, such as intermittent fasting and time-restricted feeding.

With intermittent fasting, the body switches over from glucose as its energy source to fats. This can help the health of many of the organs and systems in your body.

Time-restricted feeding involves keeping all eating to within an 8- to 12-hour period each day. Again, this has numerous health benefits.

How to Eat

Okay, so you might be thinking, "that's a bit daft." I mean, we all know how to eat, don't we? Well, we do, of course, but we all have bad habits. We will finish this chapter by introducing the idea of mindful eating.

Let's get some don'ts out of the way first though.

Don't eat stressed. This is a number one. Evolution—yes, her again—has given us tools for survival and one of those is the flight-or-fight response

I'm not going into detail on what happens, but the various chemicals released into the blood affect almost the entire body.

One part affected is the digestive system. It effectively shuts down so that energy can be diverted to fighting or running away. This shutdown reduces the nutrients that can be absorbed. Continual stress actually reduces the amount of nutrients you can take in.

Instead of metabolizing fatty acids, cells switch over to breaking down muscle, replacing it with fats.

Finally, glucose, as the instant energy source, is released into the blood. This flood can cause cravings for sugary foods.

So, relax, have a hot bath, meditate, and eat in a calm environment.

Here are a few more tips on how to eat mindfully:

> - Don't distract yourself, especially with TV. If you have conversational company, take moments to focus on your food.
> - Don't eat meals while driving or working with a screen.
> - Don't bring your worries to the table. Again, this will heighten your stress levels with all the bad stuff that it does to your body.
> - Don't eat standing up or walking. Sit, relax, and breathe. It's all to do with stress really, and the body reacts to it when this happens.

I have many French friends, and their eating habits are food centered. They take their time and spread every meal into an event rather than a refueling mission. Research shows that their physical and mental state during meals is quite the opposite of stress. (David, 1994).

Now, the be-sandalled guru has arrived, and we will consider the steps of mindful eating.

Our Jedi master informs us first that mindful eating is not only good for you but will bring back the joy and pleasure of food to your life. They suggest that you do the following:

1. **Start with your shopping trolley.** As you choose each item, consider its nutritional value, how it is packaged, and where it has come from. In doing this, you not only choose the right nutritional foods for your table, but you consider the planet, its ecosystem, and the people who have provided

you with your food. You will feel better both when shopping and eating if you know that you have made an effort to source locally with minimal packaging and have supported people through fairtrade. ("Fairtrade", n.d.). Above all, avoid the dark side: the center aisles where the processed foods lurk.

2. **Leave enough time for food preparation and cooking.** Rushing this will only lead to stress and poor results. I find that if I take an interest in learning more about cooking and how to prepare different dishes, then I enjoy the process. Often it is the highlight of the day.

3. **Sit down to your meal with an appetite primed and ready to be satisfied.** Don't be ravenously hungry, though, as that can lead to rushing your food and overeating.

4. **Focus on the quality of your food and not the quantity.** We are sophisticated humans and not pigs at the trough. Use plates that are 9 inches or less to limit your portions.

5. **Be thankful for your food.** Many people say grace or other prayers, but even those who have no religion can pause for a moment to think, with gratitude, about those involved in bringing the food to its destination in your meal. If you have company, acknowledge them out loud. Remember to thank yourself if you did the shopping or the cooking. I'm sure it's not hubris, but I often find myself looking at the feast I have prepared and saying, "You would need to get a damn good restaurant to get a meal as good as this." I know it's not as I have practiced, and that I have put a lot of time, effort, and passion into its preparation.

LET FOOD BE YOUR MEDICINE

6. **Use all your senses in enjoying each mouthful.** Smell the aromas, taste the food, and feel its texture as you eat. Do what fancy restaurants do and spend time on the presentation so that it looks awesome and good enough to eat! Try to have a mix of colors and textures. During preparation, you can listen to the sounds of cooking. Even at the table, you can hear the crunch of salads and fruits shouting their freshness to the world.

7. **Eat slowly by taking small bites and chewing thoroughly.** Too often, we gulp down food without chewing it enough to release all of its flavors. Digestion begins in the mouth, and that act of chewing releases enzymes that produce more flavors in your food.

By following these simple steps, you will find yourself enjoying your meals more. Much more than that, though, you will absorb all those lovely nutrients that you spent time preparing so much better.

Coming up, it's time to take a look at your gut and how it works. They say a good driver is one who understands how the engine works and maintains it well. Let's lift the hood and have a look.

> **YOUR GUT IS NOT LAS VEGAS. WHAT HAPPENS IN THE GUT DOES NOT STAY IN THE GUT!**
>
> — DR. ALESSIO FASANO

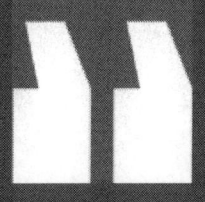

CHAPTER 6:
WHAT DOES YOUR GUT SAY?

Gut health is just health. It's where your mission to stay healthy begins. Without a healthy, well-maintained gut, your chances of the rest of you being healthy are slim.

Earlier in the text, we looked at the trillions of bacteria that live in your gut and touched on the role they play. Not only are there 1,000 species of gut bacteria inside you, but their genes are as well.

Genes are the functional instructions for making biological molecules. We have around 20,000 of these. Combined, the gut microbiota has an excess of two million.

What this means is that they have a set of tools that goes way beyond what we personally have for creating useful molecules that promote health. (Borre et al., 2014).

We will come back to them later, as their importance can't be overstated. But first, we will look at the relationship between your gut and your brain.

A Gut Feeling

There is an intimate relationship between your brain and your gut. It's actually known as the gut-brain axis and is a two-lane blacktop of communication. Signals zip back and forth to control every aspect of digestion from when to eat to when to move your bowels.

The link with our brains starts early. Research has shown that, without a gut microbiome, brain development is abnormal. (Borre et al., 2014). A fascinating experiment conducted involved implanting gut bacteria from humans suffering from depression into mice. The mice then developed behaviors similar to depression.

The bacteria that live in our guts are capable of producing many of the neurotransmitters we need, including serotonin, dopamine, histamine, and noradrenaline. Scientists are now looking at possible ways of using microbes to treat a range of mental disorders.

So, how does gut bacteria help us out? I could probably write an entire book about that alone, but here are some of the stars (Stewart, 2019):

- **Akkermansia muciniphila.** These guys strengthen your gut lining by feeding on the mucins that make up the mucus layer in your gut. This stimulates the cells lining the gut to produce more mucus. The good thing here is that a thicker mucus layer reduces inflammation. It also reduces the likelihood of obesity and protects against metabolic conditions such as insulin resistance.

- **Barnesiella.** You are really going to want this one. Not only does it help with the treatment of some types of cancer, but it prevents certain antibiotic-resistant bacteria from getting a foothold in your gut—a case of fighting fire with fire.

- ➤ **Christensenella minuta.** If you are one of those people that doesn't really put on weight, it may be due to having a horde of this lot in your gut. It's a bacteria you inherit from your parents. There are more of these bacteria in the guts of lean people compared to obese.

- ➤ **Adlercrutzia equolifasciens.** Eat soy, in whatever form, and these helpful chaps will convert some of the chemicals in the soy into equol, a powerful antioxidant that is also great on the anti-inflammatory and anti-tumor fronts. It can reduce the risk of prostate, breast, and gastric cancers.

So, let's leave it with these four. Hopefully, you are now convinced of just how important the right balance of micro-organisms in your gut is to your health.

Before we move on, let's have a quick look at the various factors that can affect the microbes in your gut, starting at the beginning.

- ➤ Your genetic makeup predisposes you to the types and numbers of bacteria species that will develop in your gut.

- ➤ If you are born by cesarean, your initial dose of gut bacteria that would normally come from proceeding through the birth canal is bypassed. Instead, you will pick up bacteria from the skin of medical professionals and anyone else in the room.

- ➤ The next step on the way to building your microbiome is breastfeeding. Mother's milk contains probiotics that infant gut bacteria thrive on. Not only that, your mother's gut bacteria make their way into her milk so that you get a good dose of microbes to get you going. (Macciochi, 2020).

- ➢ Just getting good exercise is enough to increase the diversity of microbes in your gut.
- ➢ Your surroundings also affect your microbiome. Different cultures have very different ranges of gut bacteria.
- ➢ Stuff you take in—foods, medicines, drugs, smoking, and alcohol—have an effect on your microbiome.
- ➢ Your mental state, depression, stress, and other mental conditions have an effect on your gut and the microbes living there.
- ➢ Your age also affects your gut bacteria. As you progress through the various stages of your life, hormonal and environmental changes affect your gut bacteria. Everything from puberty, menopause, moving house, or exam stress can have negative effects on your gut.

Ground Control to Major Tom

How many brains did you have the last time you looked? Of course, the answer is one. Although, there is a good case for saying that the 100 million nerve endings making up the gut's enteric nervous system is a good candidate for a second brain. These two "brains" are constantly sending messages to each other. Most of these messages are functional, controlling things like when to eat and defecate. However, bad stuff happening in your gut sends messages to your brain, and bad stuff happening in your brain sends messages to your gut. Our brains and guts intimately affect each other.

There are a few pathways between the gut and the brain. The largest nerve in your body is one of these: the vagus nerve. We have already had a look at how various bacteria in your gut can affect how you feel. In the other direction, your emotions and mental state can cause all sorts of disruption in the functioning of your gut. (Van Oord, 2019). You might be surprised to find that cognitive behavioral therapy (CBT) is more effective in providing long-term relief from irritable bowel syndrome (IBS). It even works with refractory IBS, a form of IBS that all conventional treatments have failed to help. ("Cognitive Behavioral Therapy," 2019).

That fight or flight reaction we looked at earlier is why meeting your future partner's parents for the first time can have flocks of butterflies performing aerobatics in your stomach. It's also why, when you are about to sit down for a crucial exam, you suddenly have an irresistible urge to sit down somewhere else. Yes, that's me trying and failing to make a euphemistic reference to diarrhea.

Ulcerative colitis and Crohn's disease are known to be affected by stress. As many as 70% of patients with these ailments report that their symptoms are worse during times of stress. Even yoga and mindfulness meditations have been shown to be effective in reducing the symptoms of IBS. (Kuo et al., 2015). Navel gazing works!

The Gut and Immunity

The human body is a donut! Both donuts and humans are examples of a torus. The hole is the same as the digestive tube that passes from the mouth to the anus. Looking at a donut, you can see that the hole is on the outside. You can run your finger right around it, starting inside the hole and moving to the outside, and at no point will your finger actually be inside the body of the donut.

The same is true of our digestive tube. We tend to think of it as inside us, and although it is enclosed within our bodies, the contents of our digestive tube are effectively outside our body, including food, mucus, bacteria, and stools.

If you could start with your finger on your chin and run it up over your lips, down your throat, through your stomach and gut, through your anus and back up over your body to your chin, your finger will not have lost contact with a continuous surface at any point. The bacteria living in our guts are outside of our bodies, just the same as those on our skin.

The "skin" in your gut is a thin wall of cells that prevents bacteria from getting into your body and allows things that are good for us to get in instead, most of the time. At the same time, chemicals produced by our immune system can pass through our bodies into the gut and through this layer of cells to attack harmful organisms within the gut.

In fact, most of our immune response is by this means. Our immune system is actually fighting possible infections before they actually get into our bodies. Think of the gut wall as the walls of a castle, and our immune system is firing arrows (antibodies) at potential invaders.

A significant player in this war is the colonies of bacteria living outside the castle walls in the gut. They are like the scouts or, more accurately, what the military calls "force reconnaissance;" the good old marines. Hoo-rah!

They detect potential invaders and send information back into the castle, "Get those arrows ready and start boiling the oil." At the same time, they can also attack or divert potential invaders, crowding them out or even outright killing them so that they can't reach the walls.

If our external troops don't have good eyesight or telescopes and their radio battery is run down, we don't get the quality of information that we need to prepare to fight illness.

Like a good general, you need to make sure that these troops are well cared for so that they can act as our most important line of defense—the first one.

Any army is made up of a variety of different types of soldiers: artillery, infantry, armor, reconnaissance, logistics, engineers, medical, commissary, and ISTAR (Intelligence, Surveillance, Target Acquisition, and Reconnaissance).

Without this complex set of roles—often interlocking—an army cannot function effectively.

That's your gut bacteria.

A diverse community with diverse roles. The army in your gut is fighting a constant war against infection invaders. Your gut needs lots of healthy troops, and it needs different types of troops.

If this first line of defense doesn't succeed, then the invaders breach your walls and cause mayhem within the complex city that is your body.

I'm standing down from this analogy, but keep it in your mind.

There are lots of studies into what good and bad bacteria do for our immunity. Each of them are trying to understand if more of this type or less of that type is good or bad for us.

It's a difficult study, as there are so many types, and there are a lot of interactions between them—between them and us, and between them mitigated through us. If you increase one type, then that can have knock-on effects on other types and what they do, which might affect what you are trying to measure. It's like trying to look at how increasing the number of rabbits affects the number of foxes in an ecosystem without being able to account for the eagles, pumas, and other predators.

To sum this up, listen to what Dan Peterson, assistant professor of pathology at the Johns Hopkins University School of Medicine, has to say: "'There are a lot of data right now on these relationships between changes in the microbial community and different diseases.' For example, the Human Microbiome Project has spent millions of dollars to catalog microbiome communities in people with different diseases. 'The next step is the hard step: trying to figure out all that data.'" (Fields, n.d.).

Yet, before we get all the theories from scientific investigation coming out with answers, there is one thing we can reasonably assume: Our bacteria have evolved along with us. Therefore, foods that help keep our naturally occurring microbiome as near as possible to our original paradigm are the ones we should be eating.

Those foods—the ultra-processed, for example—that were not part of that intimate mutual evolution are certainly going to upset that carefully crafted balance.

Your Gut Health Plan

Just like in politics where the aphorism is, "It's the economy, stupid," then we should have our own pithy saying that is, "It's the food, erm, gentle reader." Phew!

So, let's list the ten commandments of your health plan:

1. Eat resistant starch. This is starch that your digestive system finds difficult to break down. It passes through your small intestine and does its job in your colon. The bacteria here feast on it and produce butyrate, a fatty acid that the cells lining the colon use as an energy source, facilitating greater blood flow into your colon and keeping it healthy. It also plays a role in helping your immune system detect precancerous cells, reducing your likelihood of colorectal cancer.

2. While evidence is still being sought to conclusively show that probiotics and prebiotics are good for you, there are indications that they may be very beneficial in maintaining a healthy and diverse population of bacteria in your gut.

3. Eat fermented foods and cut down on sugar and red meat.

4. Fast, but not in a biblical sense.

5. If there are profound reasons why you need non-dietary help, then there is poo therapy. For example, for someone who has had their microbiome nuked by antibiotics and who is vulnerable to infections, then the transfer of fecal matter from a healthy individual to the patient has been shown to be very effective in re-establishing a healthy population. ("Faecal Therapy," 2013). Fear not though; pill-based versions are available, which show the same effectiveness.

6. Exercise.

7. Limit your use of non-steroidal anti-inflammatory drugs (NSAIDs). For example, most painkillers are NSAIDs. Prolonged use can damage your gut lining.

8. Try not to use laxatives. They reduce your gut microbiome. Instead, look to improving your diet with more fiber. Exercise also helps.

9. Use a probiotic after a course of antibiotics to restore your microbiome.

10. Don't use disinfectant cleaning products as often. They affect your gut bacteria in much the same way as antibiotics.

Ambrosia

So, if you want the physique of Heracles and the complexion of Aphrodite, what should you eat if the week's ambrosia delivery got diverted to Asgard by mistake?

Let's do them by food groups:

Fruits

- Mangoes
- Bananas
- Apples
- Raspberries
- Blueberries
- Pineapple

Nuts and Seeds

- Almonds

Fermented Foods

- Sauerkraut
- Yogurt
- Kefir
- Miso
- Kvass
- Kimchi
- Sourdough bread
- Kombucha
- Fermented pickles
- Raw cheese (check that it has not been pasteurized. They should be labeled raw and aged for at least six months)
- Matto
- Tempeh
- Apple cider vinegar (it should be labeled "with the mother")
- Cottage cheese

Vegetables

- Garlic
- Onions
- Leeks
- Shallots
- Jerusalem artichokes
- Asparagus

- ➢ Broccoli
- ➢ Spinach
- ➢ Brussels sprouts
- ➢ Kale
- ➢ Potatoes
- ➢ Squash
- ➢ Dandelion greens
- ➢ Ginger

Fats

- ➢ Coconut oil
- ➢ Olive oil

Proteins

- ➢ Wild salmon
- ➢ Chicken
- ➢ Trout
- ➢ Swordfish

High Fiber

- ➢ Lentils
- ➢ Artichokes
- ➢ Green peas
- ➢ Black beans
- ➢ Lima beans
- ➢ Brown rice
- ➢ Oats
- ➢ Whole meal bread

- Quinoa
- Avocados
- Chickpeas

Others

- Organic, prebiotic-, and probiotic-enhanced chocolate
- Apple cider vinegar
- Bone broth
- Collagen
- Pickles

Avoid! Avoid! Avoid!

Now we turn our attention to the delinquents of the food community; the gut-bacteria-destroying, inflammatory, and immune-suppressing bad boys. Let's line up the usual suspects and identify them.

- Sugary foods, drinks, and sweeteners
- Alcohol
- Fried foods
- Red meat
- High-salt foods
- Ultra-processed foods
- Foods containing antibiotics
- Refined carbohydrates

Notice that I haven't suggested any particular food items. It really is just a case of avoiding anything in these categories as much as possible.

Feeling Pooped?

Before I delve into this section, I would like to reassure you, my dear reader, that although this is the second time I have focused on poop, I don't have a Freudian fixation.

It is simply because the easiest way to see what is going on *in* your gut is to examine what comes *out* of your gut. You don't need any fancy chemical assays, blood tests, or invasive procedures. The evidence is right there before your eyes.

So, here is your masterclass in poop analysis.

The color, unsurprisingly, should be brown. A black stool can indicate anything from overdoing iron supplements to bleeding in your upper intestine. Pale, white, or clay-colored stools may indicate a blockage in your bile duct. Very green can indicate you ate greens—not a problem, unless your stools are passing too quickly and contain a lot of bile. Mild green, on the other hand, is fine. If your stools come out yellow, then you may have too much fat in your diet or, possibly, malabsorption. Yellow is also an indicator of possible celiac disease. Finally, red is perhaps the most alarming when you see it. It could be that you ate a bunch of red stuff. You might have hemorrhoids or bleeding in the lower intestine.

If you think you have intestinal bleeding due to frequent red or black stools, then you should get checked for possible polyps or cancer. Consult a health professional and expect to be offered a fecal occult blood test. A positive result will probably mean turning up for a colonoscopy. (Mayo Clinic Staff, 2022).

Stools should be log shaped, lengthwise and about a couple of inches, and not as a series of pellets. It should be somewhere in the region of firm and soft. Straying outside this consistency toward being too hard or a bit runny is a sign that something might not be right.

Poop shouldn't be too reluctant to leave your body. Ideally, it should vacate the premises in a minute or so and certainly no longer than 10 to 15 minutes.

If you are frequenting the smallest room in the house anywhere between every other day and two to three times per day, then that is within the normal range. Any longer, and you need to up your water intake.

The Bristol Stool Chart

Researchers at the University of Bristol in England have come up with seven categories of stool. ("Bristol Stool Chart," 2022).

1. Separate, hard, and dry small lumps that are hard to pass
2. Hard, sausage-shaped, lumpy stools that are hard to pass
3. Smooth, soft, sausage-shaped stools that are easy to pass
4. Sausage- or snake-like stools, softer and mushier than type 3, easy to pass, and can be more irregular in shape than type 3
5. Liquid stools that are soft blobs, porridge-like, or possibly small quantities of solids
6. Liquid stools that have no form with mushy, fluffy, and ragged edges; or no solid content at all
7. Completely liquid and very like diarrhea

The first two are indicative of constipation. Type-3 is the Oscar winner, especially if it is easy to pass and on the soft side. The snakey 4th type is also quite normal and should appear every one to three days.

A number two that looks like a number five indicates a lack of fiber in your diet. The runny, blobby type-6 could be mild diarrhea, and you need to look at drinking more water and some electrolyte-filled drinks.

Seven is just the runs and may be indicative of an infection.

Floating stools may contain more gas, or it could be that there is a lot of fiber.

If you are often constipated, and that means less than three movements per week, then there could be a variety of reasons, including everything from hormone changes due to pregnancy or diabetes to not having enough fiber or liquids in your diet.

Study this section and then test yourself out on the poop assessment at www.webmd.com/digestive-disorders/rm-quiz-poop.

A large part of this chapter has been a discussion of immunity. In the next chapter, we will explore the ways in which you can use food to boost your immunity.

> **THE RIGHT RAW MATERIALS CAN DOUBLE OR TRIPLE THE PROTECTIVE POWER OF THE IMMUNE SYSTEM.**
>
> — JOEL FUHRMAN

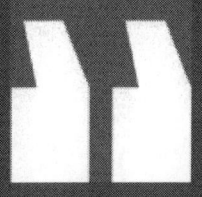

CHAPTER 7:
YOU ONLY HAVE TO LOOK WITHIN

The immune system is very complex. It keeps a record of every germ encountered in two types of white blood cells (T-lymphocytes and B-lymphocytes). This record means that these cells can quickly attack and destroy any recurrence of these bacterial infections. (Better Health Channel, 2017).

Viruses like colds, the flu, and COVID are harder to defend against, as they mutate so much between infections that it is difficult for the immune system to recognize them.

Tetanus is a bacterial infection, and the vaccination for that can be effective for up to 14 years, although it is recommended to get a shot every 10 years. The flu, on the other hand, is a virus, and vulnerable cohorts need to be vaccinated every year with the latest strain.

Your immune system has several components:

> **Lymphatic system.** The system is composed of lymph nodes that trap microbes and lymph vessels containing the clear

lymph fluid that permeates the body's tissues. The fluid also contains white blood cells that attack and kill invaders.

- **Spleen.** The spleen filters out microbes in the blood as well as old or damaged red blood cells. It is also a manufacturing hub for antibodies and lymphocytes.
- **Bone marrow.** The marrow in your bones is the blood manufacturing facility in your body, making red and white blood cells and platelets.
- **White blood cells,** which are made in your bone marrow. They move through the blood system and tissues of your body and go into action when they encounter germs or viruses.
- **Antibodies.** These lock onto antigens, which are previously encountered markers on the surface of a microbe or toxin. The antibodies effectively mark the invader for destruction.
- **Thymus.** It has two main roles: the production of T-lymphocytes and blood-filtering.
- **Complement system.** This least-known element is made up of a range of proteins that work alongside antibodies.
- **Skin.** The oil your skin secretes kills bacteria.
- **Lungs.** The mucus in your lungs is wafted up by small hair-like cell protrusions called cilia, carrying foreign particles for you to eventually cough out.
- **Gut.** Last and certainly not least, both the acid and antibodies in your gut can kill infections. Not to mention the sterling work of the microbiome.

Eating Your Way to Immunity

What you eat is critical to the good functioning of your immune system. By eating the right foods you will bring into your body the necessary balance of nutrients that keep your immune system operating at its peak.

The immune system response can be divided into two categories.

The innate system is the first responder, attacking unknown particles that enter your body. It's like the sentry at his post, firing into the dark at an unrecognized enemy that fails to provide the password. The password is the genetic signature that all our native cells possess. Like the sentry firing wildly, sometimes the target is hit, and sometimes it isn't.

The second line is the adaptive system, sometimes referred to as acquired immunity. For this to work, it has to specifically recognize an invader from a previous encounter. It's like specialized troops that have detailed knowledge from previous engagements and can choose the right weapon system to neutralize the target.

The adaptive system is a learned response. The T- and B-lymphocytes act as memory cells that are able to employ a pathogen-specific response.

Other Triggers

Apart from infections, the immune system can be triggered by a variety of other causes.

> ➤ Antigens are simply unrecognized particles that the body assumes are harmful. This can include allergens.

- ➢ Inflammation is caused by mast cells releasing histamine. Aside from pain and swelling, there is also a surge of fluid release to try and wash out pathogens. The histamine outpouring also triggers a rush of white blood cells.
- ➢ Rheumatoid arthritis, lupus, and other conditions are autoimmune diseases where the immune system mistakenly attacks our own healthy tissues.

Immune System Depression

Various factors can reduce the effectiveness of our immune systems. Two of them need very little introduction: AIDS and leukemia. Both of these severely disable the immune system to the point where it barely functions, and death results from secondary infections that the immune system can no longer fight off.

Aging is obvious on the outside; gray hair and the wrinkling of skin are the tip of the aging iceberg that permeates your entire body. As the cells in your immune organs such as the spleen, thymus, and bone marrow become more decrepit, there is a reduction in the amount of immune cells they produce. Deficiencies in micronutrients speed up the aging process.

Drinking, smoking, and pollution assault us with toxins, many of which have a deleterious effect on our immune systems.

Low-level, chronic inflammation is a side effect of obesity. Overtime this degrades the immune system too.

Stress! Once again, that busy, hectic lifestyle we all have produces things like cortisol that suppress inflammation. Remember: Some inflammation is a crucial part of our immune system, activating white cells through the release of histamine.

Poor sleep lowers the amount of a type of cytokine that we normally produce more of when we are asleep. This particular cytokine is a tool in fighting infection.

Our poor diets virtually undermine every part of our immune system from the gut bacteria diversity to the micronutrients needed by every part of our various defense systems.

The Immunological Diet

I have brought to your attention, repeatedly, how much your diet affects your ability to fight infection. A good diet provides both the macronutrients and micronutrients that our cells need to function properly. Given that our immune system is composed primarily of cells, they, too, need these nutrients.

Vitamins C and D, minerals like selenium and iron, along with amino acids like glutamine found in proteins, are essential for the production of immune cells and their functioning.

All those bad foods we mentioned in chapter six muck up your immune system while the foods you should eat enhance and nurture it. The probiotic and prebiotic foods mentioned in the same chapter cultivate the microbiome in your gut.

By focusing on good foods and shunning bad foods, you will automatically have an immunological diet.

Supplements

Sometimes supplements are necessary when there is a deficiency in particular nutrients. Remember, though, that too much of a good thing can be bad for you. Check back to chapter five and consult appendix B on what is required and what is safe.

Tea catechins and garlic may well help prevent you from catching colds and flus. However, if you do catch one, your period of suffering seems to be unaffected.

Switching on the Immune System Afterburners

Let's get down to the nitty-gritty of what you can eat and do to get your immune system functioning at its best. The key is a system of healthy living strategies.

One strategy to avoid is simply taking supplements that promise to boost the number of immune cells you have running around. Too many of these, as has been shown with elite athletes' blood doping, can result in strokes. (Wedro, 2016).

Choose the healthy route of lifestyle changes and a good diet to get your immune system up to speed. Don't make your immune system a problem by eating an unbalanced diet, smoking and drinking too much, getting irregular exercise and sleep, or raising your stress.

As we age, the efficiency of our immune system degenerates. Unfortunately, this is exacerbated by a type of malnutrition prevalent in developed countries called micronutrient malnutrition. Fighting against the aging of the immune system requires you to ensure that you have the right micronutrients.

To make sure that your immune system is working at full speed, you need to have the following micronutrients in your diet (Merz, 2021):

> ➤ **Vitamin B6.** You can get this through whole-grains, bananas, chicken, pork loin, and potatoes with skin on.

- **Vitamin C.** Good sources include tomatoes, citrus fruits, sweet peppers, kiwi fruit, and broccoli.
- **Vitamin E.** Consuming sunflower seed or oil, almonds, peanut butter, and safflower oil will boost this vitamin.
- **Magnesium.** This is available in a range of foods, including legumes, nuts, seeds, and whole wheat.
- **Zinc.** There is plenty of this nutrient in turkey (dark meat), oysters, Alaskan king crab, and beef shank.
- **Selenium.** You can find this in a variety of foods, including Brazil nuts, garlic, and onions.

There are good indications that numerous herbs may boost your immune system. ("Best Antiviral Herbs and Supplements," 2022). These include the following:

- Lemon balm
- Astragalus
- Garlic
- Licorice
- Fresh ginger
- Black elderberry
- Turmeric
- Holy basil
- Reishi mushrooms and mushrooms in general
- Oregano
- Wormwood
- Echinacea
- Elderberry

Of vital importance to your immune system is de-stressing. Too much stress in your life can seriously reduce your lymphocyte count. You should find things to do that don't involve rushing about getting things done.

We all have persistent self-talk. When this gets too critical, it increases stress levels. Move the focus of these to positive ways of looking at yourself and the world. Try singing in the shower or do some karaoke. At the very least, just listen to music. Have it on in the house or at work. Music can reduce the amount of cortisol coursing through your body.

Get out for a walk, especially into nature. As Lord Byron wrote, "There is a pleasure in the pathless woods, / There is a rapture on the lonely shore." (Poets.org, 2007). A version of this is "forest bathing." ("Forest Bathing," 2022). Hang out with your family and friends and do fun things together. No one puts on their gravestone, "I wish I had spent more time in the office."

Get into the habit of doing mindfulness meditation or yoga. Taking time to focus on yourself is key to bringing down your stress levels.

There are a lot of myths about staying warm to avoid catching colds and flus. However, the research is inconclusive. The reason why you are more likely to catch these during the winter is simply because we spend more time indoors and the virus stays airborne longer. Recently, there have been studies showing that cold-water swimming or even cold showers can have a significant effect on your immune system. One study indicated that regular exposure to cold water reduced upper-respiratory infections by 40%. (Randall, 2022). Not only does it boost your immune system; it also has a positive effect on mood. This is another way to reduce your stress. Our good friend Hippocrates made use of cold water therapy to reduce "fatigue."

Don't forget to exercise. The important factor is to make sure that it is regular. Aerobic exercise can decrease your likelihood of infections by as much as 40%. (Creveling, 2023).

Your Chemical Romance

Don't worry, despite my exhortations to try singing, I am not going to break into "Welcome to the Black Parade." Believe me, you wouldn't want to hear me sing. Perhaps I am being unfair to myself as my wife is a retired opera singer!

Nevertheless, your body is full of chemicals. We all know this. What is less well known is the complex functions that many of these chemicals perform. A significant group of chemicals, hormones, make up the endocrine system.

Regrettably, despite their vital roles within us, hormones get a bad name. Often we hear people being referred to as "hormonal," usually teenagers and women. Despite the sexist overtones, we are all hormonal. Let's take a quick look at just what the endocrine system does.

We know of at least 200 hormones that help us function. (Younkin, 2020). They mainly control the following:

- ➢ Mood (Yes. I know; the "hormonal" thing)
- ➢ Growth and development
- ➢ Sexual function
- ➢ Reproduction

- Homeostasis (meaning keeping things in balance, such as blood pressure, blood sugar levels, electrolytes, and water)
- Sleep cycle
- Metabolism
- Digestion

Although hormones are released into the blood, they are specifically targeted and will only be taken up by receptors on cell walls in tissues that are configured to accept the hormone; once the hormone is attached to these tissues, it stimulates them to perform a variety of functions. Hormones are, essentially, messenger chemicals that say, "Time to do this" or "Time to stop doing that."

The messages can be divided into two groups, the first being from endocrine glands to endocrine glands. A hormone released by one gland instructs another gland to release hormones that can affect various parts of the body. For example, the thyroid stimulating hormone (TSH) is released by the pituitary gland. Guess what it does. Yep, it stimulates the thyroid gland to release a bunch of hormones that control everything from protein synthesis and metabolic rate to neural maturation.

This brings us to the second type of hormone–hormone to organ. These hormones are communications from hormone glands that instruct various organs to carry out a function. Insulin released by the pancreas gets muscles and the liver to process glucose.

Hormones are mainly released from glands such as the pituitary, thyroid, adrenal, ovaries, testes, and hypothalamus. However, other tissues such as fat, kidneys, liver, and placenta also release hormones. Oh, and our old friend, the gut.

When your hormones get out of whack, you can end up with all sorts of nasty conditions, including both types of diabetes, infertility, obesity, thyroid diseases, and irregular menstruation.

A wide range of factors can disrupt your endocrine system. Obviously, any damage to a gland or hormone-releasing organ will have an effect, but things like gene mutations, cancers, and autoimmune conditions can mess with the endocrine system.

Balancing Your Hormones

Balancing your hormones, you are probably not surprised to find, begins with your diet. As with just about everything else we have looked at so far, variety is the key. Specifically, good fats, fiber, protein, and calories are the major requirements.

If you find that you are fatigued, gaining or losing weight suddenly, your fertility cycle is off, have PMS, painful periods, and migraines, then the cause is more than likely to be hormonal. Get tested to make sure.

The next step is to examine your diet and make sure that you are getting plenty of cruciferous vegetables such as broccoli, kale, cabbage, cauliflower, or sprouts. Your risk of estrogen-related cancers will decrease.

Hormones are built up from a variety of elements, including fats and cholesterol. The whipping boy of health—cholesterol—is needed in the production of sex hormones.

So make sure you are getting regular omega-3 through salmon, tuna, olive oil, avocados, and seeds like flax seeds and chia seeds.

In particular, avocados are a good source of beta-sitosterol, which are crucial in mediating cholesterol and cortisol levels. They also provide nutrients that affect the sex hormones estrogen and progesterone.

Lots of fiber helps to remove excess estrogens from your body. So keep eating carrots, whole-grains, beans, and squashes.

Prebiotics and probiotics, as we have mentioned so often before, help your gut and the micro-organisms living there. The gut is actually the biggest endocrine organ you have, releasing a range of hormones that control appetite and metabolism. In your diet, make sure that you have almonds, raw garlic, oats, asparagus, apples, bananas, chicory, and Jerusalem artichokes.

Eggs are brilliant at balancing hormones, especially the key ones that control appetite, including insulin and Ghrelin.

Bodybuilders are crazy for chicken breast. The reason is that they have positive effects on insulin and estrogen hormones, which is good for building muscle.

Good old quinoa is beneficial through its role in balancing female hormones. Eating this should help with pre-menstrual tension (PMT) and help you get a good night's sleep. Pomegranates prevent estrogen production and can help in the treatment of estrogen-related cancers.

Melatonin is just one of the hormones that helps regulate sleep. Cherries are a rich source of melatonin, and having a munch on these each day will help stabilize your sleep cycle.

When it comes to one of the regularly mentioned stars of our super bowl—fruits and vegetables—be careful. Many of the pesticides used on these are very bad for your endocrine system. In particular, make the following fruits and vegetables top of your organic shopping list (Eatingwell Editors, 2023):

- ➢ Strawberries
- ➢ Spinach
- ➢ Kale, mustard greens, and collards
- ➢ Nectarines
- ➢ Apples
- ➢ Grapes
- ➢ Cherries
- ➢ Peaches
- ➢ Pears
- ➢ Blueberries
- ➢ Green beans
- ➢ Peppers—both bell and hot

I'm sure that you will be relieved that many of these foods have already been promoted as being good for your health in a variety of ways, and I don't suppose you will be too surprised at the foods that are bad for your endocrine system.

The Hormone Junk Foods

So, let's list these dastards!

- ➢ Non-organic foods, especially processed and ultra-processed foods
- ➢ Factory-farmed animals
- ➢ White bread
- ➢ Dairy, especially if you find it gives you acne

- Alcohol
- Foods and drinks with added sugar
- Caffeine, specifically if it's disrupting your sleep
- Fried foods

As with previous mentions of these, the best approach is to swap out bad for good. So, replacing white bread with whole grain is one step you could take.

Finally, if you are particularly worried about hormone issues and, after seeking medical advice, you want to try a hormone diet, then you can check out these two good resources:

- balancewomenshealth.com/wp-content/uploads/2020/03/Hormone_Balance_Diet.pdf
- www.webmd.com/diet/a-z/hormone-diet

In the next chapter, I will introduce the superfoods that will help keep your gut and microbiome happy.

> **IS IT A PIZZA? IS IT A BURGER? NO, IT'S A SUPERFOOD!**
>
> ―
>
> DR. STEVE KRINGOLD

CHAPTER 8:
THE SUPERFOODS

You have probably heard about superfoods; everyone seems to be going on about them. Just another modern fad, you might think. Yet, superfoods have been around for millennia.

Quinoa was cultivated in Peru and Bolivia. It is quite a fussy crop and likes the mountains. More modern agriculture brought in more manageable crops such as potatoes, corn, and wheat. So, it fell out of fashion, and it is only relatively recently that its health properties have become noticed.

Cacao was a favored drink of peoples like the Aztecs and Incas. The Spanish invaders worked out how to make lovely chocolate, and the rest is, well, history.

No less than at least 8,000 years is how long spelt has been around. The ancient Greeks made good use of this grain.

Going on a run? Then fuel up with chia seeds, just like the Aztecs and Mayans.

Since at least 400 B.C.E., Miso has been a staple in Japanese cuisine.

Stevia was first cultivated by the Guarani of South America as a sweetener.

The Horn of Africa was home to the first cultivation of teff by the Ethiopians as much as 10,000 years ago.

Garlic probably helped the Egyptian laborers to build the pyramids and, even though Achilles is a made-up character, many Greek athletes—who were actually real—used it to fuel their endeavors in games and war.

So, don't give me that passing fad line!

Just What Is a Superfood?

There is no real category of superfoods; each of them brings something different to the table. Yet, the common features of a superfood are the general effects they have on us in the areas of good heart health, a healthy immune system, cancer prevention, reducing cholesterol, and lowering inflammation.

The general components of a superfood are antioxidants, minerals, and vitamins. All superfoods contain a lot of these, but some also have good quantities of fiber, flavonoids, and good fats.

Before we delve into actual qualifying foods, a word of caution: Do not eat just superfoods. A healthy diet is varied. Superman said, "It was Krypton that made me Superman, but it's the Earth that makes me human." (Avina, 2023). Superfoods give you that extra boost, but to stay healthy, you need the hoi-polloi of cuisine too.

Going Bananas

The very first food to be marketed as a superfood was the banana back in 1918. (Staab, 2021). So, not really a new fad. The important word here is marketing. At the slightest hint of a nutritional benefit, the food industry will start proclaiming a new superfood, with a likely price hike.

It's not rocket science, but here is the simple equation driving the industry: Superfoods = Super Sales.

One morning, you wake up, and your social media, TV adverts, and in-store marketing will be hounding your conscience with the implied message that you are letting yourself down by not rushing out immediately to buy a month's supply.

It is no accident, therefore, that a large proportion of the world's population is using food as preventive medicine.

The ancient grains mentioned above are still popular, but in recent years, a whole bunch of new, trending superfoods have been added to the list. These include the following:

- Blueberries
- Seaweed
- Moringa
- Chickpeas
- Barley
- Oats
- Matcha
- Ginger
- Turmeric
- Chia seeds

So why not just stick all of these on one plate for every meal? Apart from being singularly unappetizing, you would be fooling yourself to think you were covering all the bases.

The best approach, as I have been arguing throughout, is to aim for a well-balanced and wide variety of foods. Focus on having a super plate that will have at least some of these ingredients or superfoods.

Consider the humble blueberry. Sales of these doubled between 1998 and 2006, and sales are increasing year on year. Why?

Well, the United States Department of Agriculture (USDA) created the Oxygen Radical Absorbance Capacity database (ORAC). This instrument listed foods in order of how effective they were at removing free radicals.

Blueberries came in at number one by a significant margin. Their nearest rivals were Concord grapes and pomegranates. As number four on the charts, cranberries are only 30% as effective. ("Blueberry Juice," n.d.). Raw blueberries are nearly twice as effective.

So, what's the problem? Science has pointed its flashy laser pointer at the best of the best. However, the data is misleading, as other foods not in the database had similar and even greater values. Golden raisins, I hear you ask; what about them? Oh, they are just twice as effective as raw blueberries and don't forget blackberries, which are a stunning three times more effective.

USDA withdrew the ORAC database in 2012 due to there being no actual evidence that the antioxidant capacity resulted in major health benefits. In fact, the danger was that consumers were focusing too

THE SUPERFOODS

much on the numerical values of specific antioxidants, neglecting to account for the old adage, "Too much of a good thing is bad for you." ("USDA Says," 2012).

So, in a here-endeth-the-lesson kind of way, don't believe the hype.

Having said that, here are some superfoods to include in your diet:

- Berries, and not just blueberries
- Soy
- Teas, especially green or matcha tea
- Leafy greens
- Salmon
- Dark chocolate
- Red wine and red grapes
- Turmeric
- Barley
- Brazil nuts, and most other nuts
- Beets
- Garlic and onions
- Wheatgrass
- Spirulina
- Avocado
- Chia seeds
- Ginger
- Lentils
- Olive oil
- Mushrooms
- Whole grains
- Beans and legumes

As you can see, this list is quite extensive, and there are loads of other foods that have a good claim for being included. Again, my message is, variety is not only the spice of life; it is essential for life. Don't get bogged down in seeking the perfect combination of superfoods; don't ignore them either.

Probiotics

I have mentioned these foods before and their siblings: the mighty prebiotics, which we will look at next.

Like superfoods, these have been hyped into an industry that, worldwide, accounts for almost $70 billion dollars of consumer spending. (Wunsch, 2020).

As with my earlier warning concerning superfoods, don't make one type of food the ultimate goal of your diet. Yes, include them if they are good for you, but as part of a varied diet.

There are the main things that probiotics do for you:

- ➤ Reduces inflammation
- ➤ Improves immunity
- ➤ Keeps the cell lining of your gut healthy
- ➤ Protects against bad bacteria
- ➤ Improves digestion of nutrients

Having probiotics as a component of your diet should improve your digestive health, offsetting the damage caused to your microbiota by antibiotics. The problem with lactose intolerance is also helped by eating yogurt, for example. The bacteria used in making yogurt releases lactase, the enzyme normally deficient in lactose intolerance sufferers.

They also seem to help with IBS and, wonderfully, seem to reduce vomiting, nausea, and constipation during pregnancy. Probiotics seem to be beneficial for ulcerative colitis.

Lactic acid bacteria (LAB) reduces the enzyme production of other bacteria, which may lessen your risk of various cancers like bladder, liver, and colon cancer.

Getting plenty of probiotics during pregnancy can residue the likelihood of your child developing allergies as well.

Keeping your teeth healthy is a significant factor in affecting your life expectancy. ("Want to Know How Long You Will Live," 2015). Probiotics have been shown to reduce the bacterial plaque on teeth.

Trying to lose weight? Again, probiotics have been shown to reduce the risk of type 2 diabetes as well as reduce weight in people regularly consuming probiotics.

So, what probiotics should you be considering? The following list of foods are high in probiotics:

- Vegetables that are lacto-fermented, such as pickles
- Kombucha
- Natto
- Miso
- Tempeh
- Raw sauerkraut
- Yogurt

- ➢ Kefir
- ➢ Kimchi
- ➢ Fermented cheese like buttermilk cheese, feta, gouda, and cottage cheese ("11 types of cheese that contain probiotics," 2022)

The bacteria in your gut behave like an organ. Keeping them healthy through probiotics leads to more creation of K and B vitamins. They also turn fiber into short-chain fats, which nourish the cells in your gut lining.

Prebiotics

Let's clear up what the difference is between probiotics and prebiotics. Probiotics contain bacteria. Prebiotics are the food that keeps them going. Taken together, you have a match made in heaven.

Prebiotics are mainly resistant starches in fibers or complex carbohydrates that you can't digest. However, the bacteria in your gut can, and that's how they get energy to function and reproduce. They are consumed by bacteria in the small intestine. There are two main types of prebiotics: fructo-oligosaccharides, which contained in onions, garlic, asparagus, bananas, and artichokes; and galacto-oligosaccharides, which are contained in beans and some root vegetables.

Studies have shown that prebiotics can improve the following:

- ➢ Calcium absorption
- ➢ Immune function
- ➢ Cholesterol levels
- ➢ Brain function

They can also reduce the likelihood of some cancers, such as colon cancer, and can also prevent allergic reactions.

There are swings and roundabouts, though. Prebiotics are high in fermentables, oligosaccharides, disaccharides, monosaccharides, monosaccharides, and polyols (FODMAPs). These foods can cause IBS symptoms in some people, which may include side effects such as bloating, gas, and abdominal discomfort. On the plus side, IBDs (irritable bowel disease) such as Chron's and ulcerative colitis can be helped by prebiotics, especially fructo-oligosaccharides. (Rasmussen & Hamaker, 2017).

If you eat whole-grains and plenty of fruits and vegetables, then you will likely be getting a suitable amount of prebiotics. The following foods are good sources of prebiotics (USDA, 2020):

- Chicory root
- Dandelion greens
- Jerusalem artichoke
- Garlic, onions, and leeks
- Asparagus
- Bananas that are slightly green
- Barley, rye, couscous, and oats
- Apples
- Konjac root
- Cocoa
- Burdock root
- Flaxseeds
- Wheat bran
- Seaweed

- Mushrooms
- Chickpeas
- Red kidney beans
- Watermelon
- Grapefruit
- Cabbage

Fermented Foods

Fermented foods have been around for millennia. They are foods that have been produced using anaerobic microbes to break down sugars. Those microbes use the sugars as their energy source. However, in the process of extracting the energy from the sugars, they produce waste products. The most well-known is alcohol, but they also produce gasses and organic acids.

Be careful when selecting foods that are fermented. Make sure you pick those that say, "naturally fermented" on the label. For example, foods pickled in vinegar won't have any probiotics.

You can make your own pickled vegetables just by cutting up carrots, cauliflowers, and celery. Sterilize a large jar with boiling water. Empty the jar and then add the vegetables, a bay leaf, and one slice of chili. Top up with filtered water and just over a tablespoon of sea salt. Keep the vegetables pressed down using a cabbage leaf at the tip. Then leave the jar to ferment. The bacteria that live on the surface of the vegetables will get to work.

To make sure the process continues smoothly, do not tighten the lid. Leave enough room for the gasses produced to be released.

After a couple of days, you can test for taste, but do not double dip! You can leave it to ferment longer until you are satisfied with it.

Finally, screw the lid on tight and refrigerate. The vegetables will keep for about a month. When it's ready, add some apple cider vinegar before serving.

Fermented foods not only taste amazing, but they are also a necessary process for some foods, such as olives, which have bitter-tasting phenolic compounds if not fermented.

Eating fermented foods can reduce your risk of high blood pressure, cardiovascular disease, inflammation, diabetes, and obesity.

As with other food types we have discussed, you need to focus on varieties, as different fermented foods bring individual benefits. Yogurt helps prevent type 2 diabetes and fermented milk is good for muscle pain, for instance.

By now, you should notice a crossover in the foods listed under probiotic, prebiotic, and fermented. A lot of "good" foods serve more than one purpose.

Fiber-Rich Foods

Fiber is basically carbohydrates that you can't digest; although, as we have seen, your gut bacteria feasts on them. Fiber ends up in your colon undigested and provides most of the content for your stools.

The fiber in your diet has the following benefits:

- ➢ Helps with the regulation of blood sugar
- ➢ Lowers cholesterol

- Helps you feel full
- Reduces risk of colorectal cancer
- Reduces symptoms of constipation and diarrhea
- Reduces risk of diverticulitis
- Helps with feeding the gut biome

Depending on your sex and age, you should be consuming 25–38 g per day of dietary fiber. But there are several types of dietary fibers.

High-Fiber Foods

We have met quite a few of these foods before.

- Whole grains
- Legumes
- Nuts and seeds
- Fruits
- Vegetables

As I have mentioned before, don't fixate on specific foods. Eat a wide variety of the above categories, and you will not only get the fiber you need but a full range of nutrients as well.

Soluble Fiber

No prizes for guessing the difference between soluble and insoluble fibers. Soluble fibers can dissolve in water. They live in fruits and vegetables for the most part, and in other food sources such as Arabic gum, guar, carrageenan (found in some seaweeds), and some hemicelluloses, which are found in the cell walls of almost all plants.

Good sources of soluble fibers are as follows:

- Black, kidney, and lima beans
- Brussels sprouts and broccoli
- Avocados
- Sweet potatoes, carrots, and turnips
- Pears, apples, guavas, nectarines, and figs
- Flax and sunflower seeds
- Oats and barley

Soluble fibers lower cholesterol levels as well as slow down glucose absorption, which helps regulate your blood sugar levels.

Insoluble Fiber

Okay, the last guess counts for this too. These don't dissolve in water. Insoluble fibers are the kings of constipation. If you want easy bowel movement, then you need these in your diet:

- Amaranth
- Cauliflower
- Green peas
- Cooked prunes
- Dark, leafy greens
- Blackberries
- Nuts, especially almonds
- Beans
- Apples (unpeeled)
- Wheat and corn bran
- Whole grains

Resistant Starch

We recently met these starches. They are starches that we can't digest. Once they have made their way into the large intestine, they ferment due to the action of gut bacteria. This is their food source. Remember that fermentation is the extraction of energy from carbohydrates. Their primary role is feeding and keeping the gut bacteria healthy and diverse.

There are basically four types of resistant starches:

1. Found in grains, legumes, and seeds.
2. Contained in some starchy foods, such as green bananas and uncooked potatoes.
3. Found as a result of cooking things like rice and potatoes and then allowing them to cool. As they cool, retrogradation turns a proportion of the digestible starches into resistant starch.
4. Man-made starches that are produced through chemical processes.

So, those are the types; however, foods can contain more than one type.

Resistant starches are good for improving insulin sensitivity and lowering your blood sugar levels too. If you consume 15–30 g per day for at least four weeks, you should find a 33–50% improvement in your insulin sensitivity. (Robertson et al., 2005).

The best foods for resistant starches include the following:

- Legumes
- Potato and pasta salads

- Sushi rice
- Unprocessed whole grains

Getting More Fiber into Your Diet

We are constantly being told that we need to eat more fiber. Doing so can be achieved by following the building blocks of nutrition we mentioned in chapter four. Make sure your plate is half full of vegetables. Again, this doesn't have to be every single meal you eat, so long as you are averaging that level of diet share. Get rid of white starches and replace them with whole-grain versions.

Salads are a good way of getting more fiber as well as a ton of nutrients. Make sure you sprinkle them with seeds and chopped nuts to get that extra fiber.

Instead of drinking fruit juices, eat the fruit itself, especially with the peel on in the case of apples and pears.

Use beans and lentils in place of meat in some meals and enjoy vegetable snacks with dips like hummus.

If you are having yogurt, cereal, or oatmeal, then add some dried fruit.

Oh, and to avoid dry and hard-to-move stools, up your water intake. As you increase your fiber content, your stools will tend to become drier.

Live Long and Prosper

My good friend, Spock from Star Trek, wrote this section.

As everyone knows, I am now 160. Something tells me this might be my last year, though. Now, Vulcans like me are genetically superior to weak humans, but with the correct diet that my good friend Dr. Steve recommends, you too can enjoy living longer and healthier. Prospering is up to your own endeavors, my friend.

Anti-aging diets are clearly on the menu among human scientists, doctors, and diet professionals. (I believe that is illogical human humor). To achieve this, you must avoid fried foods, fatty meats that are saturated with saturated fats (more illogical humor), reduce your alcohol intake, and avoid ultra-processed foods. Please avoid sugary food and those with high-salt content too.

One of your human scientists, Timothy Harlan, assistant professor at Tulane University School of Medicine, said, "Poor-quality foods, like trans fats, cause inflammation, and aging is basically a chronic inflammatory state. Can you look older because you are eating crap? Absolutely." (Shaw, 2011).

Eating sugary foods and processed carbohydrates can cause damage to the collagen in your skin, resulting in wrinkles.

Aside from eating good foods, calorie restriction is often a part of anti-aging diets, including such things as intermittent fasting. You can read about this in Dr. Steve's book, *Intermittent Fasting for Women over 50: Dr. Steve's Guide for Rapid Weight Loss, Energy, Detoxification, Diabetes, and Anti-Aging.*

Some foods are very good for anti-aging, including the following:

- Green tea
- Avocados
- Berries

THE SUPERFOODS

- Dark chocolate
- Water
- Vegetables
- Walnuts
- Melons
- Beans
- Olive oil
- Tomatoes
- Soy
- Wild salmon
- Mangoes
- Oatmeal
- Lentils
- Spinach
- Grass-fed beef
- Turmeric
- Red grapes

As Dr. Steve keeps telling you: Keep your diet varied, and our advanced science concurs.

I will now hand you back to the good doctor. He assures me that he *is* a doctor and *not* a coal miner.

Thank you, Spock.

So, we have come to the end of part two. Up till now, we have been looking mainly at how foods can be used to improve your health. Along the way, we have mentioned aspects of lifestyle that are crucial.

In part three, we will take a deeper look at these.

> NO MATTER HOW MUCH IT GETS ABUSED, THE BODY CAN RESTORE BALANCE. THE FIRST RULE IS TO STOP INTERFERING WITH NATURE.
>
> — DEEPAK CHOPRA

BEATING THE INDUSTRY GIANTS

We see advertisements for medicines that are meant to heal us all the time. We see adverts for food too, but only for mass-produced products, which, 90% of the time, are bad for us. What we never see are adverts for fresh, natural ingredients – the preventative medicines that render pharmaceuticals and commercial foods unnecessary.

Both the food and the medical industries are driven by profit, and this is a big reason for our current health crisis.

My intention with this book is to help more people take charge of their own health through up-leveling their diet, and that means getting it into the hands of as many people who are looking for guidance on the subject as I can – and to do that, I'm going to need your help.

Just as adverts steer people toward the foods and medicines that are contributing to our poor health, book reviews steer people toward the information they're searching for. They act as signposts that show exactly where that information is, as well as evidence that it's helped someone else.

So, I'd like to ask you a favor: Will you take a few minutes to leave a short review?

By leaving a review of this book on Amazon, you'll show new readers where they can find the guidance, they need to take their health into their own hands and reduce their reliance on pharmaceuticals.

Simply by letting other readers know how this book has helped you and what they'll find inside, you'll show them exactly where they can find the information they need to get started.

Thank you so much for your support. We're fighting against big industries here, and we need to stick together to make sure our voices are heard, by leaving a review of this book on Amazon.

https://amzn.to/3KlT3pW

PART III
A LIFESTYLE OF CHANGE

> *Life is like riding a bicycle. To keep your balance, you must keep moving.*
>
> – ALBERT EINSTEIN

> **EXERCISE IS KING. NUTRITION IS QUEEN. PUT THEM TOGETHER AND YOU'VE GOT A KINGDOM.**
>
> — JACK LALANNE

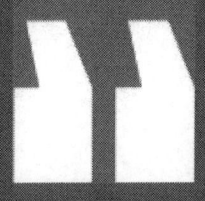

CHAPTER 9:
HEALTHY HABITS IN MOTION

You can't be healthy if you don't exercise. The best diet in the world is only part of the solution. It is the fuel for your life and using that fuel to actively make your body fitter is the second step in the journey.

There are a lot of myths about diet and exercise. One of the most persistent is that you need to do intense exercise for long periods. In fact, it is recommended that we all do around 150 minutes of moderate intensity exercise per week. (U.S. Department of Health and Human Services, 2018).

What counts as moderate intensity? Well, brisk walking is one example. Using the stairs instead of an elevator or escalator is another. Do some light weightlifting just to exercise and tone your muscles. You won't bulk out; you only get that with very intense strength training. Exercising muscle is good at burning calories. After the age of 50, you could be losing one to two percent muscle mass per year.

Oh, and dieting is hard. That's a myth we all fear. But dieting is not about giving up food. As we have seen so far, it is about eating the *right* food, not eating bad food.

Don't cut carbs; change them from unhealthy carbs to good carbs. If you cut them out, you will find yourself with low energy, tiredness, poor bowel function, and ironically, an increased appetite.

The important thing about exercise is to get into the groove, to develop a habit and a routine. Leaving it till you feel like it means you will never feel like it. There will always be some excuse.

In some ways, regular exercise can become a keystone habit, setting you up for a daily, healthy lifestyle.

Building New Habits

Before we get into how to establish good, healthy habits, we need to take a moment to consider what stage of change you are in.

Contemplation

This is where most people are. You know that you are unhappy with your diet and exercise. You also know that your health will improve if you make changes. Yet you are procrastinating due to—sometimes nebulous—barriers that you perceive. You are unsure about how you will cope with these barriers and, as a result, are actually scared of commitment. This is the hardest stage, which is unfortunate because it is the first. It is where we are most likely to fail.

In this stage, you are wired to resist (Andreatta, 2017). Over millions of years of evolution, we have evolved to be afraid of change. There are two basic psychological functions that underpin our reactions to the world: reproduction and survival. It is this last element that makes change difficult.

Back through the mists of time (Why is the weather always so bad back in time?), we liked things to stay the same. We knew where everything was and where a threat was most likely to be. If we had to move to a new place or hunt in a new environment, then we would be on edge. We would be expecting the unexpected to happen at any moment. Fear would be a dominant emotion.

This isn't just a human thing. It is a survival mechanism that developed over all the stages of evolution. (Meek, 2020).

Now, however, in our ever-changing world, it can be a major hindrance.

The secret to coping with this anxiety is to carry out a cognitive behavioral approach. Listen to your thoughts, think about them, and identify why they are irrational. Be aware that your fear is not due to the change, but to your animal brain. Reflect that you have a new brain that lets you think through things like this.

So, think!

Focus on why this change is for your benefit. Visualize what you will be like after this change and how good you will feel.

Then jump!

My good Scottish friend, who surprisingly finds golf tedious, suffered from an acute fear of heights. He cured it in his early teens at a scout camp.

Abseiling was one of the organized activities during this camp. He talks about his head spinning as they gathered at the cliff top and his overwhelming urge to run (away from the cliff, not toward it; although, in later life, he now runs toward the thrill).

As he stood there, he realized this was a big decision point in his life, a now or never moment.

He thought through, without knowing anything about CBT, why it was perfectly safe, saying things like, "Nobody dies from this, they are experts, I am no different from the thousands that have done this before."

He volunteered to go first. In effect, he jumped.

At the bottom, his hands were shaking so much it took ages to undo the carabiner. As soon as he released himself, he ran back up to have another go. Fear of heights is an innate and rational fear. (Russel, 2023).

Yet, he managed to overcome it by thinking through the outcomes.

How much easier will it be for you to think through the irrational fears associated with a beneficial change in your life?

Preparation

Okay, so you are now past the contemplation stage. You have made the decision to get on with it and stop procrastinating.

Your new brain is laughing at the animal brain.

Now, it is time to put in the steps that you need to get on with it.

Things that you will need to plan for include the following:

- ➢ **When am I starting?** There is an easy answer to that. As the old Chinese proverb goes, "The best time to plant a tree is 20 years ago. The second-best time is now." Don't procrastinate; set a time in your diary for the next day.

- ➢ **How am I going to change?** Am I joining a gym? Am I buying some weights? Am I going jogging or for brisk walks? Am I entering a mixed martial arts (MMA) competition? (Probably not the last one). List the steps you need to take. Set times in your diary. Action them and tick them off.

Remember, in this stage, you are still prone to procrastination, as your sneaky animal brain is still trying to resist. You may have to CBT the hell out of yourself again.

Action

Yes, you've made it. You are now in the phase where you have been following through on your decisions. You are feeling good about yourself and proud of yourself. You are even annoying your friends by telling them how good you feel and how they really should person-up and do the same, perhaps with a tinge of guilt at your own self-satisfaction at being better than them.

Not only that, but you are better physically. Your new diet and your new activities have your body feeling better than you can remember. Your poo is a nice healthy type two or three. (Honestly, I don't have a fixation!)

You have been in the groove for maybe six months.

As Han Solo said to Luke Skywalker, "Don't get cocky kid." (Lucas, 1977).

There is still the danger of backsliding though.

Notice that most of this is written as a visualization. Use this in the contemplation phase. Think as though you are six months down the line and how you will feel.

Maintenance

To keep your new habits going for a lifetime, you need to keep reviewing where you were, where you are now, and how much you have to lose. Set a monthly date in your diary to review your progress and set new goals. These could be further changes in your diet, increased activity, or even major lifestyle changes.

Perhaps you are now ready for that MMA challenge. Maybe you have decided to enter the New York Marathon. Who knows? Keep your options open.

Installing New Habits

All the above jokes about MMA are there for a reason. I think you probably already know that it is plain senseless to even think about doing anything extreme, arduous, or enduring from the get-go.

If you set your initial goals too high, you are setting yourself up for failure. It is more difficult to maintain a new habit if it takes a lot of time or is too hard.

Unfortunately, failure switches your emotions toward the dark depths of despair where, after more failures, you will decide that you can't change, you are not up to it, or you are a failure.

HEALTHY HABITS IN MOTION

The secret is: Start small.

Some people can ditch smoking instantly; go cold turkey. Most people get there by reducing the number of smokes they have per day or trying to have a period each day where they don't indulge in it that lengthens overtime.

Decide on one change in your diet or activity that you can easily incorporate into your routine. Each week or two, make another small change. Set these steps in your diary.

My Scottish friend that I mentioned earlier, the one who is "feart o' heights", to use his vernacular, is a physicist. He has a thing about exponentiation—what normal people know as compound interest.

If you change by one percent each day, then in 365 days, you will be almost 38 times better than you are now. Yeah, this really is a case of doing the math.

Chunk down your goals. So, if you are aiming to walk five miles a day, start off with one mile in the morning and one in the afternoon. Then add in an evening mile. Before you know it, you will be buying top-of-the-range hiking shoes, and booking a trip to Scotland to do the West Highland Way along with my Scottish friend, who will bore you with more math. I usually find that offering to buy him a dram of Lagavulin at the end of the day if he shuts up works well.

Gradual change and being patient with your progress are the way. Changing shouldn't be hard. Don't keep piling on new weights or miles to try and progress quickly. Do it gradually so it doesn't feel hard and is enjoyable. Think like the tortoise and not the hare.

You Will Fail

Yeah, while we are on the topic of walking, remember what the road to hell is paved with.

Most people find it difficult to maintain routines at the best of times. So, don't feel dreadful and, especially, don't feel a failure when you fall off the horse (How did that creature get into a walking metaphor?)

To deal with this, get back on the horse as soon as you can. (This horse is determined to stay!) Avoid slipping twice in a row, as it will then become the mode that you are in rather than just a one-off.

Think about why you failed and put in place methods for avoiding the same pitfall again. (Maybe this horse is a pit pony now).

Think ahead and list the possible reasons for failure that might lie ahead. You know yourself better than anyone, so take time to analyze the things that normally get in the way of doing things and plan for how you will avoid these or cope with them going forward. (Clear, 2018).

Finally, the guy that didn't need a horse at all—just rode around on Luke Skywalker's back for half the movie—said it all. "Try not. Do." (Kershner, 1980).

Beating Cravings

We are now going to look at another failure mechanism: cravings. We all have them. These are usually sugary, fatty, or salty foods. Maybe you are a chocoholic, for example.

These foods are often referred to as hyper-palatable foods.

Cravings are not due to being weak, having no self-control, or possessing that all-time classic sweet tooth. They are a function of how your brain works at a deep level. They are akin to but not as serious as addictions.

When you eat one of these foods, the pleasure you get—the instant satisfaction—stimulates a plethora of neurochemical signals such as cortisol, insulin, dopamine, leptin, and ghrelin.

These foods are known as comfort foods for good reason. The hormones that are released reduce feelings of stress, leading to the craving when you find your stress levels rise. What do you do? Instinctively, you reach for the thing that you have learned that chills you out. Even artificial sweeteners have this effect.

Your brain has several components that make up a reward system, the most important one being the hypothalamus. Again, evolution has developed this so that you are encouraged to seek out behaviors that reduce your stress levels.

There is no cognitive interpretation of what is the cause of the stress. The fact that your levels have gone down is all your reward centers need to say, "Do that again."

Even just thinking about a donut causes a release of dopamine, building the anticipation of the pleasure it will give you.

I mentioned addiction above. For some people, this could be a problem. Food addiction isn't agreed on by all the experts, some of whom see a difference from nicotine, alcohol, and drug addictions.

Most agree, though, that there are significant similarities. The three main similarities are as follows (Alonso-Alonso et al., 2015):

- ➢ Activation of the same pathways that trigger dopamine signals and the reward centers in the brain
- ➢ Increased tolerance overtime; to get the same hit, you need more
- ➢ Difficulty in breaking the need to use because the brain's reward centers have become conditioned to a hyperactive response

Apart from the neurochemical base for cravings, there are a number of other factors that make quitting them difficult.

Advertising

It's not on a whim that many countries have banned advertising for addictive substances such as tobacco and alcohol from sporting events, early evening TV slots, packaging, and so on.

Adverts work. They make you buy stuff, and they make you use stuff. It's why food manufacturers spend $14 billion per year on snack food advertising in the United States alone. (Ha, 2020).

To deal with the subconscious effects of advertising, notice the adverts. Analyze them from the viewpoint of what they are trying to make you do. Imagine a counter-advert that promotes the bad aspects of these foods. "Gorge on these donuts like a dirty pig until you are as fat as me and die an early death feeling nothing but regret." How's that for a tagline? Visualize the advert that you have created: a hooky tune more like a dirge than a celebration, dancing pigs, and technicolor vomit.

Use your creativity so you are not just engaging the right side of your brain as well as the fact-guzzling left.

Stress

Chronic stress can cause you to have cravings for hyper-palatable foods. The extra cortisol surging around your body stimulates your appetite and cravings.

When you are under prolonged stress, your body needs more nutrients and oxygen. You are like a car that is revving its engine even though you are going nowhere. Your body needs more food, and it is telling you to eat.

Coupled with this is the lack of time that you feel. Consequently, you go for quick fixes—ready-made meals that you bung in the microwave or eating snacks al desko.

The really bad news is that cortisol encourages the deposition of fat around the belly, which increases your risk of type 2 diabetes, breast cancer, and cardiovascular disease.

Sleep

Allied to stress is poor sleep. Often, when you are stressed, you don't get enough sleep, or you get poor-quality sleep. This can lead to fatigue during the day.

How do you deal with fatigue? Well, your body tells you to take in more energy. The quickest source of energy is sugary foods.

When you are not sleeping well, the leptin and ghrelin hormone levels are disturbed. This causes increased appetite and cravings.

Exercise

Good exercise reduces the levels of ghrelin, resulting in a reduction in appetite. At the same time, your glucagon and leptin levels are also restricted. The longer your exercise period is and the more intense it is, the greater the effects.

Effectively, you are reducing the opportunity to have appetite signals and craving urges.

Hormonal Change

During the monthly cycle, women can experience more cravings and feel less sated after eating. This occurs when estrogen levels bottom out as progesterone peaks.

The brain receptors that respond to estrogen normally leave you feeling full. So when estrogen levels are higher, women feel fuller quicker.

Estrogen restricts the release of ghrelin, which normally makes you feel hungry.

Medications

Earlier, we looked at functional medicine and its mission to find the root causes of conditions. Often, these can be found in poor diets.

As mentioned, medicines given simply to reduce symptoms often have side effects.

Your appetite can be increased by taking antidepressants such as sertraline, paroxetine, and mirtazapine, or antipsychotic drugs like aripiprazole and quetiapine.

The steroid prednisone can increase leptin resistance, causing patients to feel hungry all the time too.

Reducing Cravings

Not surprisingly, given everything that has been said before, it comes down to eating healthily.

Unless you are adhering to forms of intermittent fasting successfully, then you shouldn't have long gaps between meals. When you have a prolonged period without eating, then you feel hungrier. Duh!

The point, of course, in intermittent fasting is to feel hungry. It is something that you have to discipline yourself to do. After you have been practicing fasting for a while, your feelings of hunger reduce. Not only that, but when you do eat, you feel fuller quicker.

The reasons for this, as usual, are the levels of ghrelin and leptin. Eventually, your body releases less ghrelin, the hunger hormone. At the same time, you become more sensitive to leptin, which helps you to feel full. Keep drinking water too, as it helps you to stay full and moistens your stools if you are eating more fiber. (Lowery, 2022). And when you do eat, having a good amount of protein will help as well.

When your friends post messages showing the latest meal they have made on Facebook, don't dwell on them.

Get out of your snacking habits, like when you sit down to watch a movie or the latest installment of *The Kardashians* with a bowl of potato chips, popcorn, or chocolate. You know, those moments when you just want to self-indulge. Choose something else instead, such as an apple or banana.

Raise your dopamine levels by taking a cold shower, listening to music, walking in nature, watching your favorite comedian on YouTube, or dancing in your kitchen.

Your Binge Buttons

Binging is both emotional and psychological.

If you have irregular mealtimes, then your eating hormones get out of balance, telling your brain that you need to eat and that you still aren't full when you do.

This is where the urge to pig-out on comfort foods arises.

When we are upset, stressed, lonely, down, or angry, we have the urge to break out by reaching for something that we have learned is a source of comfort. For some, this might be alcohol, drugs, or another smoke. For many, it's sitting down with comfort foods and, well, comforting themselves. It is no accident that these salty, sweet, and high-fat foods have earned that name.

Often the urge to binge is overwhelming, as we just want to escape from our little world of pain.

To avoid binges, you need to follow the path of an addict:

> ➤ **Train yourself to identify your binge triggers.** When you experience an urge to binge, take time to analyze how you got there. Knowing your triggers is essential to getting out of binging habits.

> ➤ **Distract yourself.** In Catholic teaching, there is a thing called "occasion of sin" or *occasio peccati* if you want to impress your friends with your erudition. It just refers to

anything that can lead you down the wrong path. Along with this idea comes the simple notion of avoiding occasions of sin. Whether you are Catholic or not, it's just basic common sense. So, when you are triggered to binge, remove yourself from the situation where you normally binge. That might mean not sitting in front of the TV or lounging on the sofa scrolling through your social media. It might mean not walking past your favorite fast-food joint. The easiest thing to do is to go for a walk, preferably in nature, to recharge your emotional batteries. Or get out your needlepoint, gardening, or carpentry tools and engross yourself in something creative. Stick on some great music and dance and sing your way around the house. I know it's a risky business, but maybe cruise your way around your house in your pants and shirt like Tom Cruise.

- Jump into a luxurious hot bath or zap yourself awake with a cold shower.
- **Don't keep binge foods in your house.** It's a no-brainer. Do I need to mention occasions of sin again?
- **Phone a friend,** not to become a millionaire, but to just express how you are feeling and to receive some human comfort and encouragement.
- **Spend your money on something else** instead, like a nice massage or getting your nails or hair done.
- **Change your eating lifestyle.** Have regular, well-balanced meals and use that as the cornerstone of your life.
- **Drink water or a nice tea.** Filling yourself with something that is low-calorie helps.

Emotional eating is one of those self-feeling vicious circles: You feel upset or down. You binge eat to feel comfort. You feel guilty and powerless afterward, which takes you back to where you started—feeling bad.

Like any vicious circle, you need strategies to break out, or the process will self-perpetuate. So, sit down with pen and paper and work out what you will do to do so. Consider the suggestions above.

Activate Exercise

Want to live five years longer? Get off your butt then and move. Research shows that even moderate amounts of exercise will prolong your life and keep you feeling better during those last years.

If you exercise between 156 and 270 minutes per week, you will probably reduce your likelihood of dying within 25 years by 50%. Let's look at some of the surprising statistics that come from various studies (Crouch, 2023):

> ➤ Those of us aged between 40–69 can live longer by doing one to two minutes of exercise three times per day. Think: dancing to music around the house or taking time to jog, carefully, up and down your stairs.
>
> ➤ 11 minutes of moderate to vigorous exercise daily significantly extends life span.
>
> ➤ It helps to do that 150 minutes, but even much, much less than that is very beneficial. Going from 0–20 minutes a day has more gain than going from 80 to 100. In other words, any exercise at all is way better than nothing.

- ➤ Exercising with others has more benefits than doing it on your own.
- ➤ 7,000 steps a day over 10 years can net you between 50–70% less risk of an early death. So, walk to the shops rather than drive.
- ➤ Women over 70, in one study, who managed 4,400 steps per day lived significantly longer than those who did 2,700.
- ➤ One minute, yes, you hear right. One minute of strength exercise—30 seconds of squats and 30 seconds of push-ups—will increase your strength.
- ➤ Strength-training twice a week reduces your chances of early death by 46%.

This moderate exercise regime needs to be coupled with good nutrition. As your body changes through exercise, it needs that cocktail of protein, carbs, and micronutrients to get the benefit of the exercise.

The benefits of physical activity include the following:

- ➤ Your body feels good.
- ➤ You look better.
- ➤ You sleep better.
- ➤ You reduce your risk of disease.
- ➤ You live up to five years longer.
- ➤ Your physical condition allows you to participate in more leisure activities.
- ➤ Your mental health improves.
- ➤ You are less likely to suffer an injury doing chores.

Types of Activity

There are two main classes of physical activity. There is the one we all think of when we hear about physical activity: exercise. However, this is just a sub-group of physical activity itself. Anything you do—chores, gardening, walking the dog, or climbing stairs—are physical activities. Anything where you are moving and consuming energy is physical activity.

The real classes of physical activity, though, are as follows:

> **Aerobic.** Dancing, swimming, jogging, spin classes, tennis, and good-old walking are all aerobic.

> **Flexibility.** This includes yoga, stretching, Tai Chi, and pilates.

> **Strength.** You can get this type of activity by just digging your garden. Obviously, weights are the go-to, but strength is also increased just through push-ups, squats, sit-ups, Pilates, and working with resistance bands.

> **Balance.** Standing on one foot with your eyes closed or the classic drunk test of walking heel to toe in a straight line are good examples. Perching on a wobble board is another good example. However, any sport where you have to keep changing direction also improves balance. Balance is so important as you get older, as it reduces the likelihood of nasty tumbles.

There is no need to get the most expensive equipment around. Fitness comes with getting out of breath and putting in some resistance effort along with various stretching exercises. Keeping it simple means that you can do it more easily.

People that live to 100 have simple habits of walking, gardening, using stairs and doing household chores. Learn to use your body naturally rather than forcing yourself into uncomfortable contortions.

Beware, though, of overdoing things. It's the old problem that too much of a good thing can be bad for you.

There are obvious things like pushing yourself too hard and suffering injuries as a result, but less obvious, are the problems associated with impact exercise that can damage joints, especially as you get older.

Probably, the best exercise for all round-fitness that carries the least risk of injury is swimming.

Exercise Intensity

Believe it or not, but the simplest measure of intensity is the one used by Jean-Luc Picard. It's the Borg scale of perceived exertion. It's really quite simple. You just monitor how you feel. Are you breathing heavily, sweating more, your heart pumping harder, and are your muscles feeling fatigued? ("Borg Rating," n.d.).

So that you don't feel completely useless, the scale starts at six when you feel no exertion at all. Moderate exercise is between 11-14. From 15-20 is vigorous activity. At 20, we are really talking about sprint finishes where you are going all-out.

Multiplying your Borg rating by 10 gives you your heart rate during activities.

You can also measure exercise activity by using your heart rate and target heart rate.

LET FOOD BE YOUR MEDICINE

There is some arithmetic in this.

- ➤ Subtract your age from 220 to find your maximum heart rate.
- ➤ Your target heart rate is between 65–75% of your maximum heart rate for moderate exercise.
- ➤ For vigorous exercise, your target heart rate is between 77–93% of your maximum heart rate. ("Borg Rating," n.d.).

You can measure your heart rate by stopping your activity at points and taking your pulse or, better still, wear a device such as a smartwatch to measure it continuously. Most of these connect to apps on your phone so you can keep a regular record of your progress. If you are using exercise machines with screens, then they will normally have metal on the handles to measure your heart rate.

Then there is the fancy-sounding metabolic equivalent of task or MET. One MET is defined as the energy you are using behaving as a couch potato. Pick up a book, and you raise your MET to 1.3. If your couch goes on fire due to dropping that cigarette you shouldn't be smoking and you are forced to run, then your MET score leaps to 8 or 9.

To be clear, MET scores equate with the following:

- ➤ Sitting or lying down (less than 1.5)
- ➤ Standing or walking casually (from 1.6–3)
- ➤ Brisk walking and household chores (from 3–6)
- ➤ Digging the garden, shoveling snow, and running (above 6)

Activity Throughout Life

It might be too late now, but as a small child, you should have had about three hours of active play per day.

As you enter adolescence, you need about an hour of moderate to vigorous exercise per day.

As a younger adult, you need 150–300 minutes of moderate to vigorous exercise per week mixed with a couple of sessions of strength work.

Even as an older adult, you should keep going with the younger adult approach but include more balance exercises.

Pregnant or postpartum? Consult your doctor, but medical advice notwithstanding, aim for 150 minutes of moderate aerobic exercise per week.

If you suffer from disabilities or chronic conditions, you should try to follow the guidelines for adults, but with the cautionary guidance that you seek medical advice first. (Staff, 2018).

Always remember that with exercise, you should adopt a safety-first approach.

- Never overdo exercise by pushing your limits. You are not an Olympic athlete.
- Stop if you feel light-headed and sit down.
- Monitor your heart rate for your age as above, and do not exceed the recommended levels.
- Often is better than more. Spread your exercise across the week instead of having a burst.

➤ Make sure you are properly fueled with a good diet.

➤ Start your regime slowly and build up gradually.

You will find it easier to get into a routine if you make your exercise social. So, join a walking group or a fitness class.

Strength Training

We are going to take a quick look at this type of exercise in particular. Why? Well, for the simple reason that, as we get older, we tend to think that this stuff is for the young'uns. Going for a walk, jogging, taking the stairs, and all that mild aerobic stuff is generally regarded as the sort of thing that older people do.

You won't often hear a couple septuagenarians discussing how much they can bench. More likely they might reminisce about how much they used to bench when they were at their peak.

However, the truth is that it's absolutely essential to include strength training in your exercise routine.

As we age, we lose both bone density and muscle mass. Your muscles don't turn to fat, just to clear up one myth. However, they might as well.

Muscle tissue is much better at burning calories than fat. Depending on your individual nature, your muscle tissues can burn anything between 2.5–5 times the amount of calories your fat tissue burns, pound for pound. (Bryant, 2020).

Now, given that we naturally lose muscle as we age, what this means is that we are losing tissue that is good at burning calories. Yet, most of us keep eating as normal.

The result is that these calories that you used to burn in the muscle tissue that is now gone has to either be burned somewhere else or it turns into fat.

No prizes for guessing which.

Yes, you got it. Unless you start doing more exercise to burn off those calories, you will gain weight in the form of fat.

So, in a sense, muscle is turning into fat but in an indirect way.

Compounding this problem is that one of the ways in which we burn calories—with aerobic exercise—becomes less effective with age too. We find the following barriers:

- We can't do it as long.
- We can't do it with the same speed or intensity.
- Our cardiovascular system is less efficient.
- Joint and other damage cuts down the amount of exercise we can do.
- Our muscles are deteriorating.
- We are gaining weight in the form of fat.

What I am working up to is to get you to realize that it might just be a very good idea to slow down your rate of muscle loss so that you can keep that good calorie burning tissue and hold back on the gain of fat.

The only way to do that, and I really do mean the only way, is to do strength training throughout your life and especially as you get older.

Fortunately, we have a friend that can help. It's a giant ball of matter under your feet. Gravity is wonderful at helping us out with strength exercises.

A very simple one is to wear a weight vest when you go walking. Many of them have removable packets of sand so that you can adjust the weight. Regularly carrying an extra 10 or 20 pounds around with you will slow down the deterioration in both your bones and muscles.

When you go to the store, wear a backpack, and bring your groceries home rather than driving and having your groceries sit in a car.

Both the walking and the extra weight are good for your muscles and bones. It's very much like the weight vest, except you can eat and drink the contents.

Of course, there are weights you can use, machines at the gym, and even using the stairs is a form of strength exercise, as you are working your muscles and bones to lift something against gravity—you.

I wish I could spend more time telling you about this, but this is, after all, a book about food. Maybe in my next book!

KISS

Keep it simple, stupid. Apologies if you are offended. Walking is something we all do if we have the capability, so use that. Get out for a walk daily and try to do it with friends. You won't even notice that you are getting good quality exercise until you check your wearable device.

Brisk walking is low impact and shouldn't affect your joints. Hill-walking, on the other hand, can, especially as you come down steep gradients, which is where walking poles come into their own.

Pacing should be somewhere in the region of 2.5–4.2 miles per hour. Real benefits accrue if you get your pace above 3 miles per hour.

Build up gradually, especially if your goal is to go on a walking holiday. This applies to both space and distance. There is no need to feel sore if you increase gradually. Of course, get into the habit of walking when you can. That can be a trip to the shops or parking your car further from the mall.

If you go down the road (pun intended) of purchasing a treadmill, then start easy on it. Don't have it going so fast that you have to hold on. Build the speed up gradually during a session to allow your body to warm up. You can also change the incline gradually to increase your heart rate. Cool down at a slower pace for five minutes at the end of your routine.

If you are doing a lot of walking, then invest in good quality walking shoes. It is best to go to a sports store and get expert advice on the type of shoes you need in terms of whether you pronate or supinate, or need arch-support and flexibility.

In the sports store, you can also consult on appropriate clothing that will keep you dry but allow sweat to evaporate. I always buy my walking socks at the sports store too.

Lastly, double sock if you are doing long distances. This will reduce the likelihood of blisters.

Before we finish this chapter, it is worthwhile downloading a copy of the Physical Activity for Americans Guidelines, which you can find at the following address: health.gov/sites/default/files/2019-09/Physical_Activity_Guidelines_2nd_edition.pdf. It has all the information that you will ever need about physical activity.

Finally, journal. Keep a record of your nutrition and activity and set goals. We are so much better at sticking to things when we record and plan.

I have mentioned a few times that exercise not just promotes your physical health, but it is also good for your mental health. In the next chapter, we will turn the spotlight fully onto improving your mental health.

> THE TIME TO RELAX IS WHEN YOU DON'T HAVE TIME FOR IT.
>
> — JIM GOODWIN

CHAPTER 10:
KEEP CALM AND CARRY ON

The irony of stress is that thinking about what stresses you out stresses you out. Yet we all suffer from stress, and we all need—really need—to reduce it.

Also, every time that I see a poster with the "Keep calm" stuff, I get stressed out. That's just me, though. The message is sound.

I don't want to stress you out, but here are some alarming facts about stress:

- Three-quarters of American adults report symptoms of stress.
- Job stress affects 80% of American workers.
- No less than 49% report that stress has affected their behavior.
- Angry outbursts affect 20% of Americans.
- Mood swings affect 20% of us.
- Feeling bodily tension bothers 21% of the population.

- ➢ Around 80% of Americans were stressed by COVID-19.
- ➢ The top stressors in people's lives are
  - Money (64%)
  - Work (60%)
  - The economy (49%)
  - Family responsibilities (47%)
  - Personal health (46%)

Stress!!!

Apologies if the exclamation marks trigger a cortisol and adrenaline flood.

Let's take a look at stress itself.

Stress is the way your mind and body respond to events that cause emotional, physical, or psychological strain.

We all experience stress to some degree. Even the world's most chilled-out yogi will feel stress if they become unwell. However, we do differ in our response to the stressors in our lives, and our physical and mental ground state is a key factor in that.

If you are getting enough exercise and following a good nutrition path, then you are much less likely to have background noise of dissatisfaction. Without that plateau of well-being, you are considerably more likely to develop stress responses to triggers, and your stress experience is more likely to be chronic.

Our physical stress response is that good-old flight-or-fight, hard-wired system; the flooding with cortisol and adrenaline that shuts down digestion, increases heart rate, and increases the blood flow to our muscles.

The deal is that so long as the tiger hasn't devoured us, once the source of stress is gone, the hormone levels go back to normal.

However, our modern world leads us to live lives of near-constant stress.

Signs of Stress

The following list identifies stress signs. However, some of these signs can be due to other conditions. It is likely, though, that stress will manifest itself with more than one of the following:

- ➤ Anxiety
- ➤ Sleep disturbance
- ➤ Reduced interest in sex
- ➤ Grinding teeth
- ➤ Headaches
- ➤ Trembling
- ➤ Tense muscles
- ➤ Increased heart rate
- ➤ Feeling dizzy
- ➤ Frequent bouts of sickness
- ➤ Mood changes
- ➤ Sweaty palms
- ➤ Diarrhea
- ➤ Indigestion
- ➤ Fatigue
- ➤ Aches and pains

We can categorize these into four groups:

- **Psychological:** things like anxiety, worry, poor concentration, and memory problems
- **Physical:** including increased blood pressure, lots of infections, weight changes, lower sex drive, and disturbance of the menstrual cycle
- **Behavioral:** binging on alcohol, food, or drugs; lack of self-care; and not taking time for enjoyable pursuits
- **Emotional:** various signals such as mood swings, getting annoyed, feeling frustrated, and angry outbursts

Stress Types

Not all stress is bad. It's there for a reason after all, and that is to protect us. There are four types of stress. We will begin with the good and descend to the awful.

- **Eustress.** This is the feeling of joy that adrenaline junkies experience. We get it in sports like skiing. It makes us feel good and has a positive effect on our well-being. Eustress is a useful and beneficial stress—unlike distress, which is harmful.
- **Acute stress.** While this sounds bad, it can be positive. It is the normal fight-or-flight response when we encounter a dangerous situation. Walking home on a dark night and hearing someone behind you leads your defense system sensibly to get you ready for action.
- **Episodic acute stress.** Meaning constantly feeling that you are in situations that are threatening in one way or another.

You have moments of respite, and then something else triggers your defense system.

> **Chronic stress.** Yes, this is a case of saving the worst for last. You are in a situation that you can't escape from, such as a toxic relationship, a burdensome job with a psychotic boss, or even a childhood trauma or other trauma you can't escape from.

Stress Impacts

Ongoing stress can affect your mental, emotional, and physical health. It reduces your ability to deal with the day-to-day requirements of life, like personal care, sleep, and routine, and it interferes with your relationships, and not in a good way.

Your health also declines with more frequent incidents of illness and a greater risk of developing heart problems, gut dysfunction, diabetes, and high blood pressure.

Unexpected acute stress, like getting involved in a road rage incident, can also cause sudden death through heart attacks if you already have a heart condition.

Emotionally, you can feel drained, burned out, depressed, anxious, or frustrated. These can cause your stress levels to increase in a vicious circle.

Impacts on Eating

I'm focusing on this impact separately simply because this book is about eating your way to health.

When you are under stress, your body burns calories faster and uses up nutrients quicker. As a result, your appetite increases, and as mentioned before, you get cravings aimed at numbing out your stress.

You reach for quick food solutions both to give you the energy hit your body is demanding but also to limit the time that you spend preparing and actually eating.

You also turn to stimulants in your diet, such as caffeine, to cope with the fatigue caused by poor sleep and burnout.

The problem is that your change in eating patterns does not help you cope with stress; it occasionally masks it but, ultimately, makes it worse.

Causes of Stress

Despite the fact that our threat response system evolved to deal with predators, most of us don't have to deal with that on a day-to-day basis. So, what are the modern stressors that mess with our threat system?

- Big changes in your life, like moving house, changing jobs, bereavement, getting married, the birth of children (especially the first), or getting divorced
- A negative view of life
- Problems at work or school
- Too rigid thinking
- Unhelpful self-talk or ruminating
- Busyness and hecticness
- Relationship problems
- Inability to deal with uncertainty

- ➢ Children and family issues
- ➢ Seeing things in black and white

Remember from earlier, we are wired to resist change as a survival mechanism. Any change in your life, even those joyous ones like getting married, having a baby, and starting a new job, are major changes that will cause stress.

The Holmes and Rahe stress scale lists life events in order of greatest to least stress. Here are the top 10 (Mind Tools Content Team, n.d.):

1. Death of a spouse (100)
2. Divorce (73)
3. Marital separation (65)
4. Imprisonment (63)
5. Death of a close family member (63)
6. Personal injury or illness (53)
7. Marriage (50)
8. Losing your job (47)
9. Marital reconciliation (45)
10. Retirement (45)

The numbers after each are an estimate of how severe events are.

Further down the list with a stress value of 13 is, believe it or not, going on vacation. It's change, again, you see.

If you want to assess your current stress levels, you can have a look at the stress tool at the following address: **www.mindtools.com/avn893g/the-holmes-and-rahe-stress-scale.**

When you complete the questionnaire, only include things that are happening now or very recently. If your beloved grandfather died four decades ago, it is unlikely that this is a functioning stressor. In other words, you are not within the envelope of change.

We can also find ourselves under financial stress or if we are in an ongoing caregiver situation. These are examples of things in our lives that may not be single events but circumstances that may feel like there is no end.

Stress Overload

At what point do your stress levels, from various sources, get to the point that it is too much to cope with?

There is no definitive answer to that, as we'll all have different levels of tolerance for stress. What you might find very stressful may not affect another person as badly, and vice versa.

However, there are common factors that we all have:

- ➤ **I'm freaking out here.** Your ability to deal with your own emotions can make events worse for you. If you have trouble staying calm or are constantly losing it, then you need to deal with those issues, perhaps through therapy. It's not the stressor that is making you stressed; it's your emotional reaction to it.

- ➤ **Tales of the unexpected.** When you know something bad is coming, then you have time to prepare for it. You are getting adapted to the change before it happens. If you have a relative dying of cancer, then when death comes, you are ready for it, and, sometimes, it may even bring feelings of relief alongside grief. Needless to say, watching a loved one suffer is, in itself, a source of stress. Imagine, in contrast, how awful the stress was for the parents of children killed at Sandy Hook.

> **I want to die in my sleep**, just like my grandfather; unlike the screaming passengers in his 747. I just made that up in case you are Googling to retrospectively rubber-neck the event. A lack of control in stressful situations makes them more stressful. Take imprisonment as an example. The prisoner has no control over where he is or what he is doing and has no freedom.

> **A problem shared.** If you have a close group of family and friends that you can share your worries and fears with, then just the act of verbalizing your issues reduces stress. Someone to hold onto and hug is a great way of reducing your stress levels.

> **We're doomed,** we're all doomed, I say. Yep, pessimists are making life harder for themselves. If you see everything that happens as a catastrophe, then you will lurch from one giant stressful situation to another, thinking that each one is the worst thing ever. Having hope and a long-term positive view has that light-at-the-end-of-the-tunnel effect on you. It manages to get the stressful situation in perspective.

> **First-world problems.** If you have them, don't begrudge them; be glad that you are in a place where you can have them. A friend's daughter, going through short-term financial doldrums, moaned that she had to buy ordinary milk instead of soya. Often, you need to adopt the helicopter principle and rise up out of your situation to view the wider world and realize that things could be a lot worse.

Immunity and Stress

I have mentioned this before, but I am going to re-emphasize the fact that stress lowers your immunity levels. That's why one of the signs of stress is catching more colds and flus. That stress-sourced flood of cortisol actually suppresses your immune system.

Think about it; if you are in a fight-or-flight situation, your threat system is designed to divert all your energy and resources to fighting off an attack or running away. Any system in your body that isn't immediately required for either of those two outcomes is pretty much shut down.

Okay, that isn't a problem if you manage not to get eaten by that tiger I mentioned earlier. Once the immediate threat is gone, your body returns to normal operation.

That isn't the life we lead, though, is it? We don't have to worry about tigers. We may occasionally find ourselves in a confrontation, but our main sources of stress are due to lifestyle and tend to be chronic. So, your immune system is constantly operating below par.

Oh, and while we are on the subject of suppressed systems, can you remember where 80% of your immune system is? Sorry for springing an unannounced pop quiz on you, but I wanted to make sure you were paying attention.

Correct! Well done, you. Yes, it is the gut. Continual stress impairs the functioning of your gut, and, apart from all the digestive problems, leads to your immune system operating more poorly.

This immunosuppressive effect can happen quite rapidly. In a famous experiment, some students were assessed by both physical and psychological tests before they took an examination. Another set of students had the test done in the middle of their assessment. These students had lower T-cell counts (white blood cells) than those that were examined prior to the assessment. (Mcleod, 2023).

Take a look back at chapter six where we examined the gut-brain axis.

Taking a Chill Pill

I don't mean an actual pill, as surely by now, you realize that there are often better ways to deal with things than popping pills.

So what are the healthy ways of destressing?

Well, let's gorge ourselves on the themes of this book to begin with:

Top of the charts, unsurprisingly, is a healthy, balanced diet. All those good nutrients I introduced you to earlier in this text are essential to your overall well-being. Chapter six and its exposition of that vital gut-brain axis, just to remind you, introduced that a poor gut will affect your psychological state.

We also looked at mindful eating. The worst type of eating is that pit-stop approach where you try and get the refueling job done so that you can get on with the important task that you are laser-focused on. Wrong! The important task is your eating. It requires your focus so that you get the appropriate balance of nutrients you need. I went on, at length, about taking time to eat and appreciating your food—where it had come from and who brought it to your table—not as some new age, hippiesque, and nebulous cosmic experience man, but on a hard science approach to getting the best out of your food.

Exercise is not only a wonderful way of getting yourself to live longer, but it also reduces your stress levels. Remember: Any movement is good, so walk the dog, dance to some banging tunes, take the stairs, and leave the car at home if you can. The best stress busters are those that are rhythmic, like swimming, walking, cycling, and dancing.

Zen out, man. Get those meditation and breathing exercises going. Taking time to focus on your body and practicing self-compassion is a wonderful way of getting things into perspective and reducing your stress levels. Also, meditation has been shown to keep your telomeres from shortening, which slows down your aging. (Conklin et al., 2019). Who can resist a two-for-the-price-of-one offer?

Therapy, social support, and counseling can help you deal with underlying problems that make it difficult, if not impossible, to deal with stress too. Sort out those problems, and things might not seem so bad after all.

Get off the treadmill. No, not the one you use for jogging; that's good. I mean the one in your life where you go from sleep to work, eat, and back to sleep. Don't be that person I mentioned earlier with "Wish I had spent more time at the office" on their gravestone. Seek and achieve a balance between work and the rest of your life.

Related to that is making sure that you plan time for things you enjoy: hobbies, theater, movies, having a massage, going for a ramble in the country, chilling out fishing with whole-grain salmon and avocado sandwiches, or whatever floats your boat—which is especially important if you are fishing.

While the biblical "sleep of the just" refers to good people who are now enjoying their eternal rest, we can apply that phrase to get to bed at a decent time, satisfied that you have done your best. It's time to go through Reinhold Niebuhr's serenity prayer and realize that there are some things you can't do anything about and come to a place of acceptance. Maybe take some time to pray or meditate so that you tune out the buzz of life and find time to rest in peace. I don't mean die! No, I mean, get a good, regular sleep.

Identify and eliminate your long-term stressors. Get those things out of your life that are constantly getting you on edge.

Quickly de-stress in the moment by focusing on what your senses are sending to your brain.

Once you have identified your stressors, it is time for the four A's of stress management: avoid, alter, adapt, and accept.

1. Avoid by learning how to say no and keeping away from people that are toxic. If the state of the world is vexing you, then switch off the TV or avoid social media.

2. Alter the scene by finding compromise, balance, and expressing your needs to others. This is the opposite of bottling up your feelings.

3. Adapt or die, as the saying goes. As mentioned above, helicopter up to see your problems in perspective, and draw the boundaries of your problem. Are you knee-deep in bumper-to-bumper traffic? Well, there's nothing much to do except accept it as an opportunity to meditate or sing along to the radio. If you are stuck in a situation, make the best of it.

4. Accept those things that you can't change. You can't control the uncontrollable, so sit back and enjoy the ride

(unless my grandfather is the pilot). As in, adapt and look for the positives. Also, express your feelings so that you can more easily reach acceptance.

Meditation

It is now without question that practicing meditation is good for your overall health. It is particularly good for dealing with stress. Practicing meditation will increase your self-awareness, which is a major step in noticing what is causing you stress. You will find your negative emotions reducing and a greater ability to focus on the present at the same time.

Physically, your racing heart rate will decrease as well as your blood pressure. Added to that, the icing on the cake is an improvement to your sleep patterns.

Developing a mediation schedule can also help with a range of stress-related illnesses such as IBS. Remember: Earlier we looked at how cognitive behavioral therapy is a successful treatment for IBS. In addition to helping with this, meditation can also help reduce anxiety and depression.

There are a variety of meditation styles, and you might want to try a few until you find the one that suits you. Some of these include the following:

> ➢ **Guided meditation**, where you imagine places and imagine sensory input. One particular method involves creating for yourself an imaginary safe place, say by a waterfall under a willow. Overtime, this place will develop into a sensory and

relaxing haven. Often, you will be listening to someone taking you on a short journey and describing the scene. Typically, this is done slowly, building the world around you gradually.

- **Mantra meditation** involves the repetition of a phrase over and over and bears similarities to prayer practices in many religions.

- **In mindfulness meditation**, you focus on the moment you are in, noticing your breathing and how parts of your body feel. Your thoughts can wander, and you gently bring yourself back into focus.

- **Qi gong** involves meditation, breathing, relaxation, and even physical movement to bring yourself into harmony.

- **Tai chi** is a slow, posture-based meditation based on martial arts. The slowness of the movements requires you to focus.

- **Transcendental meditation** is another mantra-based type of meditation.

- **Yoga**, of course, is perhaps the most widely practiced form of meditation and requires focus on your movement, positioning, and breathing.

Progressive Muscle Relaxation

In many of the various meditation styles, you may find yourself being asked to focus on a particular muscle or group of muscles and notice any tensions. You then focus on relaxing that muscle before moving on to the next and repeating the process.

Breath Focus

Many relaxation techniques focus on your breathing, instructing you to breathe in a controlled fashion. Sometimes you will be asked to notice the temperature of the air as it comes in and goes out. One particularly good method is diaphragmatic breathing.

Your breathing mechanism has two features: You increase the volume of your lungs by moving your rib cage out and, at the same time, move your diaphragm down. In case you don't know, your diaphragm is a wall of muscle just below your rib cage.

In this breathing technique, you keep your rib cage still and consciously move your diaphragm down as you draw air in through your nose. Do it slowly. Then you hold that breath for a few seconds. Finally, you release the breath through your mouth by relaxing the tension in your diaphragm, again, slowly.

You repeat this focused breathing over and over as you become more and more relaxed. I practice this and find it very restful, especially listening to calming music at the same time.

Don't be surprised if you actually fall asleep during the practice—although, being asleep, you are unlikely to be surprised.

Get an Infusion of Oxytocin

A simple hug from a loved one stimulates the release of oxytocin, more commonly known as the "cuddle hormone," into your bloodstream. This hormone reduces feelings of stress and induces feelings of happiness. Hey, who would have thought? Science has proved that cuddling makes you feel good. I wonder what strange discovery they will come up with next. Group hug, anyone?

Aromatherapy

Our senses are very sophisticated, and we are all familiar with the idea of there being smells that are pleasant and others that definitely aren't.

Research has now shown that some fragrances actually help to calm you down. (Sowndhararajan & Kim, 2016).

Use Your Creativity

Paint, draw, or sketch to relax yourself. If you don't have the skills initially, then color. This might sound childish, but once again, research shows that this activity is restful, especially when coloring in complex geometrical patterns such as mandalas. (Curry & Kasser, 2011).

Long-Term Stress Relief

Many of the above are short-term quick fixes that can develop into long-term solutions with continual practice.

However, coming back to the theme of this book, the most effective means of long-term stress relief is to eat a balanced diet. This is the nearest thing to a cure-all. As we have seen throughout this book, healthy eating leads to a healthy gut, gut microbiome, better mental health, a more effective immune system, and a reduction in stress.

Without this component in your life, then other stress reduction techniques will be less effective.

Some supplements can also help you relax if taken over a period of time, including melatonin, B vitamins, the amino acid L-theanine, and an herb called ashwagandha. You should be able to get all of these at a health-food store or online.

Self-Talk

They say the first sign of madness is talking to yourself. No, it's not. We all do it, maybe not out loud, but inside, we often have a conversation with ourselves or even with others, especially if we have fallen out with a loved one.

Self-talk is not harmful unless you find yourself in a loop, ruminating about a problem.

Have you ever found yourself saying negative things to yourself? Stupid? Failure? Those are the self-talk moments we notice most. What you need to do is practice self-compassion and talk to yourself like a loving parent to a child. Point out all the good things about yourself. Often, we get angry with ourselves because we have behaved in a way that is inconsistent with our core beliefs. Instead of berating yourself for that failure, compliment yourself on having those fundamental, noble standards that you hold yourself to.

If you have nodded off while reading this, you can skip the next chapter. All the stress reduction methodologies in the world won't help much if your sleep is poor. Sorting out your sleeping habits, though, requires knowledge. So, despite what I said, you do need to read the next chapter.

> SIR, IN MY HEART, THERE WAS A KIND OF FIGHTING THAT WOULD NOT LET ME SLEEP.
>
> — WILLIAM SHAKESPEARE

CHAPTER 11:
LULLABY OF A HEALTHY LIFE

In most of Shakespeare's work, sleep is a metaphor for death. In Frank Herbert's *Dune*, Paul Atreides says, "Sleep is the little death that brings total oblivion." (Herbert, 1965).

It is little wonder that writers across the centuries have likened sleep to death, as when we are sleeping, we are not conscious of ourselves except, somewhat, in those periods when we dream.

We spend somewhere between a quarter and a third of our lives in this state of virtual non-existence. Why?

In our hectic world, it has become a badge of strength for people to boast, especially in business, how little sleep they manage to get by on.

It is a foolish attitude and masks the underlying problems of lifestyle with bravado. Unfortunately, this harmful attitude is promoted by CEOs claiming how much they get done by reducing the time they are asleep.

We need sleep. It is a necessary part of life. If we don't get enough or our sleep is poor, we suffer mentally and physically.

Now, this is a book about food being your medicine, so we are not spending forever on this, but it will help if you understand some of the science behind the function of sleep.

The Science of Sleep

So, despite my intro about lack of consciousness, our brains are actually quite active during sleep, just not in a way that we are aware of, mostly.

Sleep, as you may already know, is divided into rapid eye movement (REM) and non-REM phases.

When you nod off at night, you enter the first stage of sleep, which is a halfway world between being awake and being asleep. During the second stage of light sleep, your heart rate and breathing settle down, and your body temperature reduces because you are not using your muscles.

Deep sleep is the third and fourth stages of your sleep cycle. We now believe that it is during deep sleep that your mind orders memory and learning.

Then you enter the REM phase. During these periods, your brain waves are similar to those when you are awake. As the name suggests, your eyes move constantly beneath your closed eyelids. What most people don't realize is that you become paralyzed as you dream. So, all those movies with people thrashing about as they dream have missed the point.

These steps are repeated maybe four or five times during the night. With each repetition, the amount of time you spend in deep sleep gets shorter.

Why Do We Sleep?

The exact reasons are still not fully understood, but one theory relates to how we are constantly receiving input from the world around us. In order to cope with this input, our brain needs to be able to adapt to new information and experiences. This adaptability is often referred to as "brain plasticity."

During sleep, that plasticity is re-invigorated, allowing us to process memories and new learning. Without good sleep, we can't learn or remember information.

On top of this, like any metabolic system, our brain cells produce waste products. Getting rid of this happens more efficiently during sleep.

Despite not fully understanding why we sleep; we do know quite well what happens when we don't get enough sleep.

Without good sleep, you can find symptoms of depression increasing. You run the risk of a number of problems, including migraines, seizures, high blood pressure, reduced immunity, greater susceptibility to infections, hormonal problems, developing pain, cardiovascular disease, and diabetes. ("What Happens to Your Body When You Don't Get Enough Sleep," 2022).

Sleep deprivation can lead to cognitive symptoms such as slowed down thinking, a shorter attention span, poor memory, poor decision-making, and mood changes.

During sleep, much like our highways, the repair team comes out in the form of hormones and proteins to rebuild damaged tissues.

Sleep and Circadian Rhythms

We all have an internal clock that is managed by a bunch of cells in the hypothalamus. If you really must know, they are known as the suprachiasmatic nucleus (SCN).

The SCN controls the release of the hormone melatonin and, guess what? That stuff makes you sleepy. Melatonin normally peaks between midnight and dawn. There is another bump in levels in mid-afternoon. *Hola, siesta*!

These are the times when we are supposed to be asleep, naturally.

In addition to melatonin, the circadian rhythm responds to light levels. When the light levels are changed in relation to our internal clock, it takes time for the clock to reset. It's this disturbance of light that is at the root of jet lag, and many travelers and even shift workers benefit from light therapy. (Simran, 2023).

As light levels decrease, melatonin production increases, preparing you for sleep. This is why some people suffer from seasonal affective disorder (SAD). Due to long periods of darkness in winter, some people end up overproducing melatonin.

Learning to Dance with the Sandman

The first step in getting a good night's sleep is knowing how much you need. For adults, this is generally between 7–9 hours per night.

As you get older, it generally takes longer to fall asleep, from about 16 minutes at age 20 to 19 minutes at 80.

We'll look at this in more detail later.

As a result of spending less time in "repair" sleep, you age faster. Getting a decent night's sleep is one way of reducing your aging rate.

So, now that we have established the basics, to get a good night's sleep, do the following:

- **Reduce your caffeine intake** and don't have any close to bedtime.
- **Quit smoking.** Yes, sleep is yet another thing that tobacco is bad for.
- Your bedroom should be used for sleeping and, well, the other thing we get up to when we are not alone in bed. **Avoid having screens,** whether it is the TV, laptops, cell phones, and so on.
- **Keep the room cool,** between 18–20 degrees Celsius.
- **Good exercise** during the day promotes good sleep at night.
- **Silence is golden**, and it pretty much helps with sleep too. If there is a lot of noise around, then you should use earplugs.
- **Having a nightcap drink** may help you nod off, but it results in poorer quality sleep.
- **Have a regular schedule** with a fixed bedtime and your alarm set for the same time each morning. Remember to keep the gap between the two to around 7–9 hours.

- **Don't work late,** as you won't be able to shut off thoughts about what you have done and what you still have to do. Make sure you have a relaxation or entertainment gap between work and bedtime.

- **Cut the illumination.** The blue component of light reduces melatonin production, so using red filters or dimming lights will help to prevent this. This is related to the sky being blue during the day but turning reddish as the sun sets. Due to the way that the spectrum of light is scattered by the atmosphere, blue light is scattered more at sundown than the red end of the spectrum. (May 2022). Our inner clock is responsive to the decrease in blue light as dusk approaches. Computer screens don't follow a circadian cycle, but you can install one from ustgetflux.com/

- **Use the meditation and breathing exercises** we looked at earlier to relax your mind and body when you are in bed. At least half of insomnia is caused by stress or emotional issues. So, follow the techniques in chapter 10 to reduce your stress.

- **If you wake during the night, don't look at the clock,** as it may cause anxiety and prevent you from getting back to sleep. Oh, and that's another reason to avoid alcohol and caffeine. As diuretics, you might find the need to visit the bathroom during the night. Don't try to *get* back to sleep, as that will build anxiety. Instead, focus on relaxing. If necessary, read for a while.

- **Be outside** in the sun for at least 30 minutes each day.

Improving the Quality and Duration of Your Sleep

There are three factors that relate to your sleep cycle:

> **Sleep intensity**, which is the percentage of your sleep that is deep sleep or REM sleep. This isn't really under your control, as you are in the land of nod when this is going on. You can help your body by making sure you have a good diet, controlling the light levels in your bedroom, and getting exercise.

> **Length of sleep.** Normally, you will wake up when your body decides that it is time. If you are beholden to an alarm, then you may wake up before you are truly ready. Make sure that you go to bed at a time that ensures you have an average of 8 hours of sleep per night. Gradually go to bed earlier each night until you find yourself waking up naturally before your alarm sounds.

> **Timing.** In a way, this should be number one! It is incorporated in number two, as you need to find the best time to go to sleep at night. You can use trial and error to determine what works for you.

Recovering From Lack of Sleep

Don't worry too much if you have a night where you only manage to get very little sleep. Just make sure you sleep longer the next night, and your body will take care of adjusting your REM and deep sleep durations.

However, don't get into a habit of having short sleeps followed by long sleeps, as this will lead to sleep deprivation overtime. In fact, at age 60, you would need to sleep for 10 hours to get the same quantities of these phases as a 20-year-old gets in 7.

Getting Your Engine Running in the Morning

Fill up your water supplies with a big glass of water. During your sleep you have been losing water through breathing and possibly sweating without any intake. Your body may well be slightly dehydrated.

Remember that our sleep control is governed by sunlight too, so get outside. Interior illumination does not have the same spectrum as actual sunlight. Before cameras and cell phone cameras became sophisticated, the white balance had to be manually adjusted when moving from indoors to sunlight to compensate for this difference. Unfortunately, cell phone manufacturers can't upgrade your light-sensing gear. So, get outside and get some sunlight as early as you can.

The Two-Minute Technique

Anyone that has driven long distances will have experienced feeling drowsy. If you are sensible, you pull over and have a nap rather than drive into an on-coming 18-wheeler.

Now, if you can imagine being a jet pilot, drowsiness is even more of a problem, and they can't pull over.

To avoid rapid unscheduled disassembly (RUD), as SpaceX chooses to describe a rocket exploding, the U.S. military developed a technique that helps their pilots fall asleep quickly. On the ground, I hasten to add.

It has four steps, and you may be familiar with most of the process, as they are used in many relaxation methods.

1. Relax your facial muscles and concentrate on each little group: tongue, jaw, lips, and eyes.
2. Release shoulder tension by dropping them down as low as you can, comfortably. Then relax your arm muscles in sequence—upper right, lower right, upper left, and lower left.
3. Breathe out slowly and relax your legs, beginning with your thighs and working down to your feet.
4. Clear your mind for 10 seconds, and then do one of the following:

    a) Visualize lying in a canoe, looking up at a calm, clear blue sky. (Don't worry about the blue light, as it is imaginary and not physical).

    b) Visualize lying in a black velvet hammock in a completely dark room.

    c) Repeat "don't think" over and over for about 10 seconds.

Now, don't expect this to work the first time. It takes practice over weeks for this to really switch on. Once you are in the groove, you can phone up the air force and ask for a spin in an F-16.

There is a stand-off between stress and sleep. Stress makes it difficult to get quality sleep, and poor sleep is a cause of stress.

It isn't really a chicken-and-egg situation, though. You need to reduce stress first. Once you have that under control, then your sleep should improve, and the stress associated with that will decline.

So, we are about to draw down the final curtain on this book. In the next chapter, we will look at the medicinal uses of plants.

> **HERBS ARE THE FRIEND OF THE PHYSICIAN AND THE PRIDE OF COOKS.**
>
> — CHARLEMAGNE

CHAPTER 12:
NATURE HAS THE ANSWER

Herbalism has been around for forever. People have been using plant-based medicines since before we recorded history. Physical evidence found in a 60,000-year-old Neanderthal's grave in Northern Iraq indicates the use of herbal cures in their culture. (Sharma et al., 2021).

The earliest recorded mention of herbal use goes back to China in 2800 B.C.E. (Sturluson, 2014).

In Western civilization, the ancient Greeks weighed-in in about 400 B.C.E. with our hero, Hippocrates. They were followed by the Romans and then Arabic culture. Perhaps the most famous proponents during the development of herbal cures in the west were Avicenna at around 1100 C.E. and Paracelsus at the beginning of the sixteenth century.

Despite this long history of efficacy, modern Western medicine does not make much use of herbal cures. When was the last time your doctor prescribed you ginseng tea to reduce inflammation? This is despite nature kindly providing us with the origins of some drugs such as aspirin (willow tree bark) and morphine (poppies). The World Health Organization (WHO) has declared that 11% of our essential and basic medicines originate from flowering plants. Given that we also get medicines from non-flowering plants, a significant part of our medicine base is originally plant derived. (Pavid, 2021).

In this chapter, we will look at how herbals can be used to treat conditions. A word of warning, though: Don't become the "physician that heals thyself," to paraphrase the bible.

While many herbs are effective, for example, St. John's Wort has been shown to be as effective in mild depression as the modern SSRIs (Ng et al., 2017), they can also have side effects and can interfere with other medicines such as, blood thinners, some cancer treatments, some pain medications, and birth control treatments. (Klemow et al., 2011).

So, the object of this chapter is to raise your awareness of what various herbs can do. It is not the purpose of this chapter to turn you into a self-prescribing pseudo-doctor. If you have a condition or ailment, you need to discuss options, including herbs, with a medical professional.

Above all, don't fall into the trap of listening to so-called experts on social media or YouTube. Certainly not those who decry everything about modern medicine and promote the use of natural remedies only based on so-called evidence they have accumulated, which is not rigorous in its nature and instead, is the product of confirmation bias.

Plants That Heal

Plants contain active ingredients just like those listed on a packet from a pharmaceutical company. You have met some of these already, such as flavonoids.

Let's not beat about the bush (oh dear, sorry) and instead, start to look at some important herbs. Some of them are old friends we have met before.

- **Echinacea** can be used to stimulate your immune system to fight infection. It is often used for the treatment of herpes, fever, and boils.
- **Dong quai** can help with PMT, menopause, and high blood pressure.
- **Garlic** reduces the risk of heart disease by means of lowering cholesterol and other blood fats. It is also a good antiviral and antibiotic and can be used in the treatment of colds, flus, sinusitis, and many other respiratory conditions.
- **Ginger** is good for nausea that you might suffer from as a result of motion or morning sickness.
- **Ginkgo biloba** helps with poor circulation and tinnitus.
- **Ginseng** is great for fatigue, and it can also lower blood cholesterol and blood pressure. But if you use too much, it can actually raise blood pressure.
- **St. John's Wort** or *hypericum perforatum*, as mentioned above, is just as effective as antidepressants for the treatment of mild depression. It is also good for anxiety and insomnia. Just remember my warning above.

- **Chamomile** is a bit of an all-rounder and is used for anxiety, relaxation, wound healing, and fighting inflammation.
- **Feverfew.** Well, with a name like that, no prizes for guessing that it is used to treat fevers. It can also be used to treat migraines and arthritis. It should not be used alongside NSAIDs or anticoagulants.
- **Goldenseal** is often used to treat diarrhea and eye and skin irritations. In high doses, it is toxic.
- **Milk thistle** can be used to reduce cholesterol and treat liver conditions.
- **Valerian** might be good for helping you sleep. The evidence is not conclusive, but some studies indicate its effectiveness.
- **Turmeric** can help with joint arthritis, and some dermatological conditions and has both anti-inflammatory and anticancer properties.
- **Evening primrose oil** can help with dermatitis, polycystic ovary syndrome, multiple sclerosis, breast pain, diabetic neuropathy, and eczema.
- **Flaxseed** can reduce blood pressure, reduce the risk of colon cancer, and reduce obesity. It has powerful antioxidant and anti-inflammatory properties. It is also one of the safest herbal supplements.
- **Tea tree oil** helps with mild acne, athlete's foot, small wounds, insect bites, and dandruff. It has good antimicrobial properties.
- **Grape seed extract** is good for lowering cholesterol and helps circulation in the legs. Recent studies also indicate

that it can prevent cancer and also halt cancer cell growth. (Kaur et al., 2009).

- **Lavender oil** is good for anxiety, getting to sleep, migraines, lowering blood pressure, and has anti-inflammatory benefits.

You can find information on a full range of herbs at: www.nccih.nih.gov/health/herbsataglance.

Side Effects

Just as with pharmaceuticals, herbal medicines contain powerful ingredients. It's why they work. These ingredients can have side effects. These include asthma, allergic reactions, nausea, vomiting, headaches, and diarrhea.

Just because these chemicals come from a natural source doesn't mean that they are any safer than the chemicals found in synthetic drugs.

Fighting Cancer with Flowers

Instead of bringing your loved one a bunch of decorative flowers, serve them up in a salad.

Okay, that was a test. Just checking to see if you were thinking, "Didn't he just say to consult a professional and not self-prescribe?"

However, the people of Madagascar have long used the Madagascar periwinkle to treat diabetes. In the 1950s, researchers discovered that the plant contained significant anticancer chemicals.

From this discovery, the drugs vincristine and vinblastine were developed. In 2018, due to sequencing the genome of the periwinkle, the exact enzymes needed to produce vinblastine were identified. This should lead to the drug being synthesized. At the moment, one gram of vinblastine requires the harvesting of 500 kg of the plant. (Pavid, 2021).

The search for wonder drugs in the plant kingdom has accelerated in recent years. It is quite possible that there are new wonder drugs out there that have yet to be discovered. Nature, as it often has, can point the way to new treatments.

Unfortunately, that super-wonder-drug plant may have become extinct. It is difficult to count the number of species that become extinct as we might not have discovered a plant before it dies out. Of the ones we know, about eight die out every three years. Three years ago, 571 species had been identified as becoming extinct since 1750. However, this is one of those tip-of-the-iceberg things. The real number may be 10s or 100s of times more. "The extinction rate [is] 500 times greater now than before the industrial revolution." (Carrington, 2019).

This rapid increase in extinction is primarily due to deforestation. Yet another reason, other than climate change, to keep our forests.

Herbal Supplements

If you take a plant-based medicine internally, then it is a supplement. These can be in powdered form, chopped up, in capsules, or as liquids. You can consume them in teas, tinctures, powders, or pills.

They are not monitored by the FDA, as they are treated as foods and not medicines. As a result, the quality and standards of these products can be very variable. Also, they cannot make medical claims. So, for example, a St. John's Wort supplement cannot claim to treat depression, but the packet can say it "enhances mood."

Again, I can't emphasize how important it is to consult a medical professional before ingesting supplements to treat yourself.

Garbage Out

We've come full circle from our introduction, where we looked at the old saying garbage in, garbage out.

However, you might now be worried about all the junk that you have been eating. In this final section, we will look at how to get that garbage out.

Detoxification

Have a word with a medical professional about starting a detox diet. The diet itself is very similar to the healthy plate approach. Drink about six to eight glasses of filtered water per day. To avoid stocking up on BPA, use glass containers rather than plastic. Then it's on to eating organically grown fruits and vegetables, skinless chicken, whole non-glutinous grains, fish, eggs, nuts, and green tea.

Do not eat any foods that are processed.

Remember that your body has various systems for detoxing, and you can help them along by drinking plenty of filtered water, getting at least five servings of fruit and (cruciferous) vegetables per day, and eating fiber, lean protein, and naturally fermented foods. It's why we have evolved these big livers and the pair of kidneys we have. Even the process of sweating removes toxins.

Cleansing is a process that is sometimes used. It is more focused than the detox above and often involves just drinking fruit and vegetable smoothies for days to weeks.

There are also colon cleanses that involve flushing out your bowel with water and additives such as herbs or coffee. The scientific evidence for this is thin, however.

Elimination diets, which we met before, can also be used as a cleansing process and are good for identifying allergies and intolerances.

Risks of Cleansing

Colonic irrigation can run the risk of bowel perforation, introducing infections, dehydration, and electrolyte imbalance. In fact, dehydration and electrolyte imbalance is a risk in all forms of cleansing.

Many juices are high in oxalate. The problem with this is that oxalate lowers your ability to absorb calcium. If the juices you are drinking are unpasteurized, then you also have another pathway for introducing infection.

Simple Detox Methods

Time for a short list of effective detox methods that are part of your normal healthy lifestyle:

- ➢ **Exercise.** This gets your blood moving, your lungs working, and your sweat pouring. All of these are pathways for getting toxins out of your body.
- ➢ **Sauna.** Yep, sweating again.

- ➤ **Dry brush skin.** By doing this, you unclog pores to let sweat flow more freely.
- ➤ **Consume fiber.** We looked at how fiber is important in ensuring your body is healthy at length several times. Specifically, though, stools are a means of removing toxins.
- ➤ **Deep breathing.** It gets more oxygen into your system as well as ensuring air flushes muck out of your lungs.
- ➤ **Hydrotherapy.** Take a five-minute hot shower followed by a 30-second cold shower, and then get under your duvet for 30 minutes.
- ➤ **Destress.** Stress releases toxins. Use the advice in chapter 10 to achieve this step.
- ➤ **Drink two quarts** of filtered water each day.
- ➤ **Protect your liver.** You can do this by consuming burdock, milk thistle, and dandelion root. Also, cut down or eliminate your alcohol intake.
- ➤ **Vitamin C.** This vitamin aids in the production of glutathione, which is needed for removing toxins.
- ➤ **Sleep.** Just follow the advice in chapter 11. Your body detoxifies better when you are asleep.
- ➤ **Processed foods.** Eliminate sugary, fatty, and ultra-processed foods. Not only are you introducing toxins directly, but these also facilitate the production of other toxins in your body.
- ➤ **Prebiotics and Probiotics.** Eat these regularly.

There you are. It's not complex, and most of it will be right there in your healthy diet anyway.

CONCLUSION

So, time for last words. In reading this book, you have taken the first step to ameliorating conditions you might have, reducing the likelihood of illness, improving your overall well-being, and living longer.

You were motivated to read this book because you know something needs to change. You maybe even had a notion that your diet was at the root of any problems you might have.

What's the next step?

Plan.

Remember that road to hell? It's all very well having good intentions, but if you don't plan, you will procrastinate and, ultimately, fail to change.

So, the moment you encounter that final period at the end of this book, do your planning. That is step one.

Remember the old adage that no battle plan survives contact with the enemy. The enemy, in this case, is your day-to-day life, friends, family, work, and everything else, but especially you.

CONCLUSION

If you fall by the wayside, don't wallow in the muck of despair and self-recrimination. Get back up immediately, dust yourself off, get back on that horse we left grazing in chapter nine, and trot off into your metaphorical sunset, which, if you have been learning, will be much further away than before.

What, you're still here? That was the final period just there. Okay, here's another one, but I'm not giving you anymore. Get planning! Apologies, that was an exclamation. Here's the period.

Don't forget to refer to appendix A & B resources!

ONE LAST THING...

As you step forward into a new phase of health and vitality, you're in a unique position to spread the word.

Simply by sharing your honest opinion of this book and a little about your own journey, you'll show new readers exactly where they can find the health guidance they're looking for.

Thank you so much for your support. Together, we can make the world a healthier place.

>>> Click here to leave your review on Amazon for the eBook version.

http://amazon.com/review/create-review?&asin=B0CD7P4QVJ

APPENDIX A

Healthy eating isn't complicated. It isn't about counting calories or macros. If we just think about a typical nine-inch plate, then we can quickly visualize just how much we should eat of the various wonderful health-supporting foods. ("Healthy Eating Plate," n.d.).

What's on Your Plate

Your healthy plate should contain:

- **Half a plate of vegetables and fruits.** These give us dietary fiber as well as minerals and vitamins. Eating a variety of these will reduce the risk of cancer, strokes, and heart disease.
- **A quarter plate of whole grains.** Stick to whole-grain products such as brown rice, whole meal foods (bread, pasta, wraps, biscuits, noodles, and oats. These unrefined foods reduce the risk of diabetes and heart disease.
- **A quarter plate of lean meats or other good sources of proteins,** including fish, seafood, poultry, dairy, nuts, beans, tofu, legumes, and eggs. We need protein in our diet to create body tissue and repair damage to tissues.

LET FOOD BE YOUR MEDICINE

In addition to these three basic principles, it is important to do the following:

- ➤ **Drink water,** especially with meals instead of sweetened drinks. This will reduce your calorie intake, keeping your teeth healthy, and helping with weight control.

- ➤ **Healthy oils.** Use soy, olive, sunflower, peanut, and canola oils in your cooking. These contain unsaturated fats. Remember that many vitamins are only soluble in fats (A, D, E, and K). We absorb these better when they are in higher-fat foods. (Fletcher, 2020). However, avoid creamy or sugary dressings, as they contain a lot of calories.

- ➤ **Cooking methods.** Reduce the amount of oils and fats by choosing to boil, steam, roast, or grill your food. If you want to fry, then use an air fryer. (Ryan, 2023). Remember, though, that you should try to cut down on fried foods as much as possible.

Sample Diet

So, what should you eat? A good start is to follow the typical Mediterranean diet. Research over the years indicates that it has the greatest health benefits. It includes things such as unsaturated fats in olive oil, seafood (especially oily fish), fruit, vegetables, cereals and whole grain breads, nuts, peas, beans, lentils, seeds, avocados, balsamic vinegar, yogurt, rice, feta, and parmesan cheeses, chicken, lean-cut grass-fed beef, and a moderate amount of red wine. (Johnson, 2022). However, the fats that you consume on this diet are omega-3 and monounsaturated fats, avoiding the saturated fats found in meats and butter.

APPENDIX A

Whole foods are also part of the diet that avoid trans-fatty acids.

Sample Menu

Breakfast

- Toasted whole grain bread
- Almond butter
- Apple slices
- Goat cheese

Lunch

- Tomato and roasted red pepper soup
- Baby carrots, hummus, and whole-grain crackers
- Yogurt with grapes and strawberries
- Afternoon snacks
- Walnuts
- Dried apricots

Dinner

- Halibut sauteed in olive oil with lemon and thyme
- Couscous with tomatoes, parsley, and chickpeas
- Asparagus with olive oil and black pepper
- Salad of mixed greens, olives, tomatoes, cucumbers, and parmesan cheese shavings, dressed with olive oil and balsamic vinegar

The above reflects the traditional eating habits of most people. However, research indicates that we should follow a regime of intermittent fasting. I covered this in my other books.

Healthy Foods for a Quick Meal

The easiest way to make sure that you are able to put together a meal without too much planning or fuss is to have a good selection of healthy options in your store cupboard.

Many of the items listed below can also be used as snacks, such as dried fruits and seeds. We will put "snack" next to those. However, remember that they are also vital in your meal planning. For example, you might snack on dried apricots, but they can also be used in tagines.

- **Olive oil, sesame oil, canola oil, coconut oil, and ghee.** These all help your body absorb antioxidants, certain vitamins, and minerals. (Spritzler, 2023).
- **Coconut milk.** This may improve heart health. It is rich in phenols (antioxidants), helps with weight loss, and fights infection. (Eske, 2023). It is used widely in Thai cuisine.
- **Plant-based milks.** These contain less saturated fats than animal milk and don't contain hormones or antibiotics. Look out for those that are fortified with vitamins and minerals as well as omega-3. (Kaff, 2020).
- **Sea salt.** This has a wide range of benefits over refined salt. (Retno, 2017). However, bear in mind that too much salt in your diet is bad for you and can lead to high blood pressure, among other things. The recommended daily intake is less than a teaspoon. This can be deceptive though, as many foodstuffs especially canned and processed, contain high levels of salt. (Van De Walle, 2018).
- **Dried pasta.**

APPENDIX A

- **Red wine, apple cider, and balsamic vinegar.** Recent research has shown that apple cider vinegar may have anti-inflammatory, antioxidant, antidiabetic, and healthy heart properties. (Benisek, 2022).

- **Fermented foods** such as pickles, sauerkraut, raw cheese, probiotic yogurt, and kimchi. (Marcene, 2021). These can help reduce blood sugar levels and inflammation as well as improve overall digestive health. (Weaver, 2021).

- **Dried herbs** such as basil, oregano, rosemary, bay leaves, and thyme.

- **Dried and canned lentils and beans** such as cannelloni, pinto, black bean, and chickpeas contain nutrients such as fiber, B vitamins, iron, and magnesium.

- **Dried fruits** such as apricots, plums, raisins, and mangoes. (snack)

- **Seeds** such as pumpkin, sesame, and sunflower. (snack)

- **Nuts** such as pine, almond, pecans, and walnuts. (snack) Along with dried fruit and seeds. You can combine these with salads, yogurt, your own trail mix, and smoothies.

- **Whole and canned tomatoes.**

- **Tomato paste.**

- **Canned fatty fish** like tuna, salmon, herring, and sardines.

- **Miso paste.**

- **Honey, agave, and maple syrup.** These are a better source of sweetening in cooking compared to refined sugars. However, all sugars should be limited in use. Honey contains anti-inflammatory chemicals, antioxidants, and antimicrobial qualities. (Nordqvist, 2023).

- **Maple syrup.**
- **Olives** (black and green).
- **Artichoke hearts, capers, sun-dried tomatoes, and roasted red peppers.**
- **Grains,** including buckwheat, spelt, oats, barley, brown rice, quinoa, and millet. Be creative. You can use them in soups, salads, pilafs, breakfast bowls, and more. They are a good source of fiber, B vitamins, manganese, and magnesium.
- **Rice, couscous, and risotto.**
- **Bottled sauces** such as salsa, tamari, apple, pesto, curry, and apricot chipotle.
- **Vegetable and chicken broth and stock.**
- **Onions and garlic.** These can help with reducing mental decline, and risk of heart disease, cancers, and diabetes. (Ducharme, 2019).
- **Eggs.** These contain antioxidants and a wide range of vitamins and minerals. They may help in reducing the risk of heart disease and other ailments. (DoctorNDTV, 2019).
- **Full-fat yogurt** will likely keep you safe from high blood pressure, heart disease, and diabetes. ("Is Full-Fat Milk Good," n.d.).

In addition to the above, which are mainly fresh, raw, or single-ingredient foods, there are now a huge number of healthy snacks that contain many of the good foods we have discussed in the book—everything from protein bars to vegetable crisps. (Tucker &

APPENDIX A

Todd, 2022). Be aware, though, that many of these are high in salt or sugars.

Eating for Specific Conditions

There are eight principles of food and health that you should try to follow. These are:

1. The combined activities of all food substances make up nutrition. The whole is greater than the sum of the parts.
2. Taking vitamin supplements on their own is not the path to good health.
3. Plants are the best source of nutrients. There are very few nutrients that are better supplied by animal sources.
4. Diseases caused by genes function when an environmental factor switches them on. In other words, a major environmental factor is nutrition, and what you eat can cause these genes to be expressed and result in disease.
5. Good nutrition can offset the negative effects of harmful chemicals.
6. Nutrition that helps prevent disease also helps to stop the disease or even reverse it.
7. Nutrition that is very effective in treating one chronic disease will also support your general health.
8. All aspects of our health are affected by good nutrition.

Healthy Bones

Maintaining good bone health requires a mixture of vitamins and minerals. Principal among these are calcium and vitamin D. The main source of calcium are dairy products such as milk and cheeses. However, those on a vegan diet or who have an allergy or intolerance can obtain calcium from a variety of other foods, such as canned sardines or salmon (with bones), dark green vegetables, calcium-fortified juices, soy milk, and tofu. ("22 Calcium-Rich Foods," 2022).

Calcium goes hand-in-hand with vitamin D, which helps the body absorb calcium. The main sources of the vitamin are sunlight and milk. Fortunately, some of the alternative sources of vitamin D are the same as for calcium: canned salmon and sardines, for example. ("Food Sources of Vitamin D," n.d.).

Magnesium works alongside calcium too. You can find magnesium in foods such as sunflower and pumpkin seeds, lentils, almonds, whole-grains, spinach, and tofu.

Vitamin K helps increase bone density for people with osteoporosis and reduce the incidence of fractures. The best food sources are green leafy vegetables. ("Food Sources of Vitamin D," n.d.).

Finally, the mineral boron reduces the amount of urinary excretion of calcium and magnesium. You can find this mineral in apples, prunes, raisins, tomatoes, soy, peanuts, honey, dates, and seafood. ("The Top Boron," n.d.).

Healthy Brain

The brain needs choline to produce a neurotransmitter (acetylcholine). The best foods are eggs, peanuts, soybeans, potatoes, bananas, tomatoes, oranges, oats, milk, lentils, sesame and flax seeds, cauliflowers, and whole wheat bread. ("Choline," 2022).

APPENDIX A

Omega-3 fatty acids are good for the fatty tissues in the brain. The best source is fish, such as mackerel, herring, salmon, tuna, and halibut. Walnuts, pumpkin seeds, and flax seeds are also good sources. (Irvine, 2021).

Vitamin E is an antioxidant that protects the fatty tissues of the brain. You can find it in foods such as hazelnuts, olive oil, red bell pepper, spinach, sunflower oil and seeds, and tomato puree. (Joseph, 2023).

B vitamins help to lower levels of certain chemicals related to dementia. They can be found in brown rice, quinoa, oatmeal, and lentils. (Seow, 2023).

A lack of zinc in your diet can lead to cognitive decline. It can be found in red meat, liver, egg yolks, seafood, soybeans, sesame seeds, and sunflower seeds. (Ruggeri, 2022).

Antioxidants reduce the damage to the brain caused by free radicals. There are many foods that have antioxidant chemicals, such as vitamin C in oranges, small red beans, blueberries, red kidney beans, and prunes. (Kloss, 2022).

Decreasing Inflammation

The omega-3 fatty acids we mentioned above also help with reducing inflammation.

There is an enzyme known as COX2, which is responsible for inflammation. This enzyme can be inhibited by consuming vitamin C in citrus fruits, onions, soy, garlic, and green tea. (Super User, 2005).

Turmeric is well renowned for a variety of health properties, not least of which is combating inflammation, especially in arthritis. ("7 Health Benefits of Turmeric," 2021).

Healthy Heart

Oils from fish and olive oil help to reduce inflammation, which is a risk for cardiovascular disease.

Nuts and seeds help to reduce LDL cholesterol, reducing the risk of blood clots. Almonds and pumpkin seeds are particularly good. ("11 Foods that Lower Cholesterol," 2021).

The B vitamins mentioned previously also have a role in reducing cardiovascular disease. Specifically, they reduce homocysteine levels.

Antioxidants are a means of reducing free radicals that can damage the heart. The same foods that provide antioxidants for brain health also help the heart.

Soy helps to reduce inflammation and LDL cholesterol. Tofu, soybeans, tempeh, miso, and soy nuts all help.

Aspirin is often prescribed to reduce platelet clumping. However, cocoa has the same effect. Dark chocolate is the best source. (Swanson, 2006).

In essence, much of what we have mentioned in this appendix already is the basis of the Mediterranean diet.

APPENDIX B

This appendix will cover the following food groupings:

- Carbohydrates
- Proteins
- Whole grains
- Fats and cholesterol
- Salt and sodium
- Vitamins and minerals

However, you will soon see that there are many overlaps between these groups. For example, a healthy source of carbohydrates is whole grains.

Carbohydrates

These are usually labeled as the villain in many diets. However, there are good carbohydrates that should form part of your diet. Forget about how many carbohydrates you eat and concentrate on the quality of the carbohydrates. They are the primary source of energy that our cells need to keep functioning. Sugars, starches, and fibers are all examples of carbohydrates. Of these, sugar is the most easily absorbed, next to starchy foods like bread. They need to be broken down into sugars by the digestive system before they can be absorbed. You may even remember a simple school experiment: chewing a piece of bread until you taste sweetness. This is due to the ptyalin in our saliva. This enzyme starts the process of breaking down the starches we eat into sugars so that the body can absorb them. (Vedantu, 2023). It is worth noting that all the foods we have been discussing in the book get broken down by acids and enzymes so that they can be absorbed.

Healthy sources of carbohydrates include whole-grains, fruit and vegetables, and beans. As with most foods, the more carbohydrates are processed, the less healthy they become. The actual carbohydrate molecules don't change but processing them removes minerals and vitamins as well as introduces additives that can be harmful. Remember: Fresh is best.

Proteins

Proteins are needed by the body for growth and repair. They are a macronutrient like carbohydrates. This means that their molecules are very long. They're typically broken down into amino acids for absorption. As with carbohydrates, the source of protein can determine whether it is good or bad for you. Our body has thousands of different types of proteins (including enzymes), which are constructed from 20 amino acids. Out of these 20, most can be produced by the body. However, there are a few that we can only get through food. We must eat proteins that can be broken down into these.

Most people associate protein with meat. However, meats also come with high quantities of saturated fats and sodium. Worse still are processed meats such as sausage and bacon. (Cassetty, 2019). In addition to the saturated fats and sodium in raw meat, they often have additives such as nitrates. It hasn't yet been identified just how much processed meat is unhealthy, but once or twice a month is reckoned to be okay.

The best sources of proteins are eggs, almonds, chicken breast, cottage cheese, Greek yogurt, milk, lentils, lean beef, fish, quinoa, pumpkin seeds, shellfish, tofu, soya, beans, and peas. (Kubala, 2022).

Whole-Grains

It would not be an overstatement to say that whole grains are a wonder food. Grains that are refined remove the outer bran layer of the grain as well as the inner germ layer. Both of these contain a range of nutrients that are very beneficial to health and can reduce the risks of a number of conditions by a significant margin. Certain types of cancer, type 2 diabetes, heart disease, and inflammatory diseases are all reduced in risk by eating whole-grains. Your general bowel health also improves, and you are less likely to suffer from constipation.

If you look back at the healthy plate, you will see that a quarter of the plate is whole grains, underlining just how vital these are. Ideally, you should consume about six ounces of whole grains per day.

The fiber in the bran of whole grains helps waste pass through your digestive tract. However, it also slows down the absorption of sugar into your bloodstream, which reduces the risk of sugar spikes. These spikes can cause lethargy and hunger. As a result of the hunger episodes, you may find yourself eating more than you need to. A slower release of sugar into your bloodstream maintains a more constant level of sugar in your blood. ("Carbohydrates and Blood Sugar," n.d.).

Be aware that many foods labeled with whole grain may be misleading. ("Whole grains," n.d.). Look for the following on the label:

- The whole-grain stamp; supported by the industry.
- Whole grain is listed as the main ingredient.
- Added sugars are not in the top three ingredients.
- A value for the carbohydrate-to-fiber ratio of less than 10:1.
- The word "whole" in front of any grain.

Some grains contain the protein gluten. There are many people that have intolerances or allergies to gluten. It can even cause diseases such as celiac. However, there is no evidence to suggest that gluten is harmful to people that don't have these conditions. Gluten has prebiotic properties and is good for your gut. You should only follow a gluten-free diet if you have a specific condition. ("Gluten," n.d.).

Good sources of whole grains include spelt, barley, rye, buckwheat, bulgur, brown rice, sorghum, and oats.

Fats

You probably regard fats as a bad actor in your diet. While that is true for some fats, it is not the case for all fats. Fats are an essential component. Many vitamins are only soluble in fats. To get these, you need to consume foods containing fats.

There are three classes of fats:

- **Trans fats.** They are not as common in foods as they once were simply because these are the worst of the classes of fats. They are found mainly in processed foods and should be avoided, as even small amounts can lead to disease.
- **Saturated fats.** These are found in dairy products, red meat, and even coconut (90% saturated) and palm oil. ("Fats and Oils," n.d.). They are not as harmful as trans fats, but they should be consumed sparingly.
- **Unsaturated fats.** Both monounsaturated and polyunsaturated fats are much less harmful than the other classes. If you eat moderate amounts of these, they are good for your health. They contain vitamins A, D, E, and K and are important for a functioning immune system and a healthy brain. They are also a source of energy. They are found in many oils, such as olive, canola, corn, sunflower, peanut, and rapeseed. They are also found in nuts and seeds and a range of vegetables. ("Fats and Cholesterol," n.d.).

Vegetables and Fruits

Going back to the healthy plate, vegetables and fruits should make up half of it. As the old saying goes, "An apple a day keeps the doctor away." (Ajmera, 2020).

Fruits and vegetables are very beneficial to your overall health, reducing blood pressure, lowering the risk of heart disease, some cancers, and eye and digestive problems. As with whole grains, they also slow the rate of absorption of sugar. Eating a range of fruit and vegetables ensures that you are taking on board a wide variety of nutrients. ("Vegetables and Fruit," n.d.).

It's worth being aware of the nine classes of fruits and vegetables ("Classification of Vegetables," 2016):

- Brassicas
- Fruits
- Gourds and squashes
- Greens
- Fungus
- Roots and tubers
- Pods and seeds
- Stems
- Baby vegetables

You should try to include a selection from all of the categories in your diet.

Another consideration is the color of the fruits and vegetables you eat. When I was a child, we were encouraged to "eat our greens." Nowadays, the sensible approach is to include a rainbow of colors in your diet. ("Should You Eat a Rainbow," 2017). Every color of vegetable or fruit comes with a range of nutrients that are essential to keeping your body healthy.

Salt and Sodium

Salt is bad for you! That is what we all tend to hear from a variety of sources. But this isn't true. Salt is not only good for you, but it is also necessary for your body to function. (Martel, 2023). Marathon runners like me know this only too well. During a marathon, runners sweat a lot and lose salt from their bodies. (Machowsky, 2017). If they don't drink liquids containing salts, then they run the risk of cramps, headaches, nausea, and a whole range of other symptoms.

You may not be a marathon runner, but your body still needs salt, specifically the sodium in the salt for your cells to function properly. It is also needed for nerve impulses, relaxing muscles, and maintaining the body's water balance.

You need about 500 mg of salt per day. Most of our foodstuffs contain salt. As a result, you need to be careful about how much you add to dishes. It is recommended that your daily intake should be less than a teaspoon. Most Americans consume, on average, 3,400 mg of salt daily. (Dorfner, 2016). This is almost seven times what our body needs.

When you are looking at your salt intake, a good place to begin is the labeling on foodstuffs. It will indicate either the amount of salt or the amount of sodium. Sodium makes up 40% of salt, and about 75% of the salt you consume is hidden in your food. (Brazier, 2017).

On every label, you will be able to see exactly how much sodium or salt it contains. You can multiply any sodium content by 2.5 to get the salt equivalent. By doing this, you should be able to get an idea of how much salt you are consuming. Note that on most foodstuffs, the label will tell you the overall content but also give you an indication of how much salt there is per serving.

There are quite a few foods that are particularly high in salt and should be eaten sparingly. For example, a serving of breaded shrimp can have as much as 800 mg of salt. Fresh shrimp is only about 100 g. (McCulloch, 2023). Other foods and snacks like crisps, soups, ham, pizza, sub sandwiches, canned vegetables, processed cheese, and dried meats contain large amounts of salt.

So, what are the downsides of too much salt in your diet? Going from the least damaging to the most: headaches, kidney stones, osteoporosis, high blood pressure, enlarged heart muscles, kidney disease, stroke, stomach cancer, heart failure, and heart attack. (Haghighi, 2021).

Vitamins and Minerals

You have probably thought that vitamins and minerals are a good thing in your diet and may even take supplements. They are not just a good thing; they are essential. Without the right amount of vitamins and minerals, many of your body's systems won't function. We have just looked at a specific mineral, which is salt, as it has significant health problems if we take too much. With other vitamins and minerals, it is not so easy to take too much unless you are taking far too many supplements.

A good example of a mineral that tends to be overconsumed is iron. It is needed by the body. For example, the red color of your blood is due to iron. Sometimes people need to take iron supplements, as their bodies are low. However, taking too much can be very bad for you. The iron itself is toxic as a chemical, and our bodies carefully regulate how much is absorbed through a hormone called hepcidin. Over a long period of taking too much iron, it is possible to cause fatal damage to your brain and liver. (Arnarson, 2023).

The difference between minerals and vitamins is their nature. Minerals are inorganic, whereas vitamins are organic in origin.

APPENDIX B

Cooking can cause vitamins to break up, but it won't affect minerals.

In all, there are 14 vitamins and 16 minerals (including sodium) that the body needs to function normally. For each of these, there is a recommended daily amount that you need to take in, and for most, there are limits on how much is good for your body. ("Vitamins and Minerals," n.d.). In particular, you need to be careful with how too much of one type of vitamin or mineral can affect another. In appendix A we saw that vitamin D is needed to help with the absorption of calcium. However, the absorption of copper can be severely reduced by too much vitamin C. (Harvard Health, 2018).

So, what do they all do?

Vitamins

- Vitamin A is good for vision, prostate, bone growth, the immune system, and reducing the risk of lung cancer. It's an antioxidant. Recommended daily amount (RDA): 900 mcg. Upper limit per day (UL): 3,000 mcg. Too much can be harmful to bones.

- B1, thiamine converts food to energy and provides healthy skin, muscles, brain, and nerves. RDA: 1.2 mg. UL: not known.

- B2, riboflavin converts food to energy and provides healthy skin, hair, blood, and brain. RDA: 13 mg. UL: not known.

- B3, niacin converts food to energy and provides healthy skin, blood, brain, cells, and nervous system. RDA: 16 mg. UL: 35 mg.

- B5, pantothenic acid is good for converting food to energy, making fats, neurotransmitters, steroid hormones, and hemoglobin. RDA: 5 mg. UL: not known.

- B6, pyridoxine lowers risk of heart disease, helps the production of niacin and the neurotransmitter serotonin, helps the production of red blood cells, and plays a role in cognitive and immune function. RDA for people who are 31 to 50 years old: 1.3 mg; for people aged 51 or older: 1.7 mg. UL: 100 mg.

- B9, folic acid helps create new cells, helps prevent brain/spine birth defects (therefore, necessary for all women of childbearing age), reduces the risk of heart disease, and colon and breast cancer. RDA: 400 mcg. UL: 1,000 mcg.

- B12, cobalamin lowers risk of heart disease, helps the production of new cells, breaks down fatty acids and amino acids, protects and aids the growth of nerve cells, helps the production of red blood cells and DNA. RDA: 2.4 mcg. UL: not known.

- Biotin converts food to energy, makes glucose, breaks down some fatty acids, and promotes healthy bones and hair. RDA: 30 mcg. UL: not known.

- C ascorbic acid lowers the risk of some cancers, protects against cataracts (for this, it can be taken as a long-term supplement), helps make collagen, serotonin, norepinephrine, helps the immune system, and is an antioxidant. RDA: 90 mg; (smokers add 35 mg). UL: 2,000 mg.

- ➢ Choline helps make acetylcholine (neurotransmitter), helps with transporting and metabolizing fats. RDA: 550 mg. UL: 3,500 mg.
- ➢ D calciferol helps maintain calcium and phosphorus levels in the blood, strengthening bones, and forming bones and teeth. RDA for ages 31–70 is 15 mcg: for ages 70 and older, it's 20 mcg. UL: 50 mcg.
- ➢ E alpha-tocopherol is an antioxidant that protects vitamin A and some lipids, and may prevent Alzheimer's. RDA: 15 mcg. UL: 1,000 mcg.
- ➢ K phylloquinone and menadione helps blood clotting and may prevent hip fractures. RDA: 120 mcg. UL: not known.

Minerals

- ➢ Calcium is good for building bones and teeth, assisting muscle function, blood clotting, and nerve impulse, hormone secretion, enzyme activation, and blood pressure. RDA: 1,200 mg. UL: 2,500 mg. A high calcium diet can lead to prostate cancer.
- ➢ Chloride is a component of stomach acid and balances body fluids. RDA: 2 g. UL: not known.
- ➢ Chromium helps with the activity of insulin, maintains normal blood glucose levels, and releases energy from glucose. RDA: 35 mcg. UL: not known.
- ➢ Copper helps make red blood cells and assists with iron metabolism and the immune system. RDA: 900 mcg. UL: 10,000 mcg.

- Fluoride is needed for bone formation and reduces dental cavities. RDA: 4 mg. UL: 10 mg. Excessive amounts are harmful to children.
- Iodine is needed in the thyroid hormone. RDA: 150 mcg. UL: 1,100 mcg.
- Iron is needed for red blood cells (hemoglobin), body chemical reactions, and the making of amino acids, collagen, neurotransmitters, and hormones. RDA: 8 mg, but for women aged 19–50, it's 18 mg. UL: 45 mg. Vegetarians need to supplement.
- Magnesium is needed for body chemical reactions, muscle function, blood clotting, regulation of blood pressure, bones, and teeth. RDA: 420 mg. UL: 350 mg for supplements.
- Manganese helps bone formation, the metabolism of amino acids, cholesterol, and carbohydrates. RDA: 2.3 mg. UL: 11 mg. Too much can cause liver damage.
- Molybdenum is part of a range of enzymes. RDA: 45 mcg. UL: 2,000 mcg.
- Phosphorus helps maintain healthy teeth and bones and the conversion of food to energy. Part of DNA, RNA, and phospholipids. RDA: 700 mg. UL: 4,000 mg.
- Potassium helps to balance fluids, steady the heartbeat, aid nerve impulses, assist with muscle function, and reduce blood pressure. RDA: 4.7 g. UL: not known. High-dose supplements may cause toxicity.
- Selenium is an antioxidant that regulates thyroid hormones. RDA: 55 mcg. UL: 400 mcg.

- Sodium helps to balance fluids, aid nerve impulses, and assist muscle function. RDA: 2,300 mcg. UL: not known. Too much causes high blood pressure and a range of ailments.

- Sulfur helps with the creation of protein structure and in building healthy skin, hair, and nails. RDA: unknown. UL: unknown.

- Zinc helps with the formation of enzymes, new cells, and proteins; aids the immune system; enhances taste and smell, progresses wound healing, and releases vitamin A from the liver. RDA: 11 mg. UL: 40 mg. Vegetarians need to take supplements.

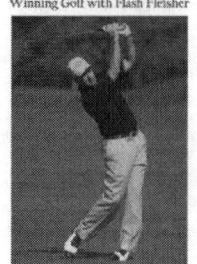

OTHER BOOKS BY DR. STEVE KRINGOLD

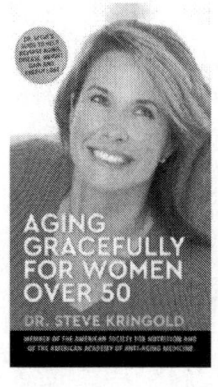

https://amzn.to/3rPtasf

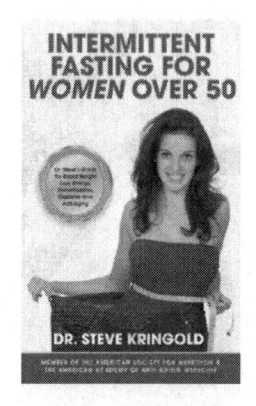

https://amzn.to/44JHwcc

https://amzn.to/475OZ7f

REFERENCES

Agostino, J. (2022, November 30). *Database indicates U.S. food supply is 73 percent ultra-processed.* Food Tank. https://foodtank.com/news/2022/11/database-indicates-u-s-food-supply-is-73-percent-ultra-processed/

Ajmera, R. (2009, November 6). *The effects of poor nutrition on your health.* Livestrong.com. https://www.livestrong.com/article/31172-effects-poor-nutrition-health/

Ajmera, R. (2020, July 6). *An apple a day keeps the doctor away - fact or fiction?* Healthline. https://www.healthline.com/nutrition/an-apple-a-day-keeps-the-doctor-away#other-options

Albert Einstein: (2015, March 13). *Life Is like Riding a Bicycle.* Big Think. bigthink.com/words-of-wisdom/albert-einstein/.

Alexander, L. (2023, January 24). *Your ultimate guide to healthy grocery shopping.* Health Digest. https://www.healthdigest.com/986364/your-ultimate-guide-to-healthy-grocery-shopping/

Alonso-Alonso, M., Woods, C. S., Pelchat, M., Grigson, S. P., Stice, E., Farooqi, S., Khoo, S. C., Mattes, D. R., & Beauchamp, K. G. (2015). Food Reward System: Current Perspectives and Future Research Needs. *Nutrition Reviews, 73*(5), 296–307. https://doi.org/10.1093/nutrit/nuv002

American Heart Association Editorial Staff. (2018, April 18). American heart association recommendations for physical activity in adults and kids. https://www.heart.org/en/healthy-living/fitness/fitness-basics/aha-recs-for-physical-activity-in-adults

American Heart Association Editorial Staff. (2021, November 1). How much sodium should I eat per day? https://www.heart.org/en/healthy-living/healthy-eating/eat-smart/sodium/how-much-sodium-should-i-eat-per-day

Andreatta, B. (2017). *Wired to resist: the brain science of why change fails and a new model for driving success.* 7th Mind Publishing.

Anthony, A. (2022, October 16). *Fast food fever: how ultra-processed meals are unhealthier than you think.* The Guardian. https://www.theguardian.com/science/2022/oct/16/ultra-processed-food-unhealthier-harder-to-avoid-than-you-thought

Arnarson, A. (2023, March 27). *The dark side of iron - why too much is harmful.* Healthline. https://www.healthline.com/nutrition/why-too-much-iron-is-harmful#TOC_TITLE_HDR_4

REFERENCES

Avina, A. (2023, January 22). *DC comics: 12 most inspirational quotes from superman.* CBR.com. https://www.cbr.com/superman-most-inspirational-quotes/

AZ Quotes. "TOP 25 IMMUNE SYSTEM QUOTES (of 139)." *A-Z Quotes*, www.azquotes.com/quotes/topics/immune-system.html.

Banks, P. (2015, June 5). *The auto-repair industry discriminates against women. So I quit my engineering job to become a mechanic.* The Washington Post. https://www.washingtonpost.com/posteverything/wp/2015/06/05/the-auto-industry-discriminates-against-women-so-i-quit-my-engineering-job-to-become-a-mechanic/

Baxter, S. (2012). *Stone Spring: The Northland Trilogy.* Ace.

Benisek, A. (2022, December 29). *Apple Cider Vinegar.* WebMD. https://www.webmd.com/diet/apple-cider-vinegar-and-your-health

Bergers, E. (2016, December 16). *1.6: agriculture and the neolithic revolution.* LibreTexts Humanities. https://human.libretexts.org/Bookshelves/History/World_History/Book%3A_World_History_-_Cultures_States_and_Societies_to_1500_(Berger_et_al.)/01%3A_Prehistory/1.06%3A_Agriculture_and_the_Neolithic_Revolution

Better Health Channel. "Immune System." *Vic.gov.au*, 2017, www.betterhealth.vic.gov.au/health/conditionsandtreatments/immune-system.

Blueberry Juice Tops The ORAC Antioxidant Chart. (n.d.). https://www.wildblueberries.com/?pressreleases=blueberry-juice-tops-the-orac-antioxidant-chart

Borg Rating Of Perceived Exertion. (n.d.). https://www.physio-pedia.com/Borg_Rating_Of_Perceived_Exertion

Borre, E. Y., O'Keeffe, W. G., Clarke, G., Stanton, C., Dinan, G. T., & Cryan, F. J. (2014). Microbiota and Neurodevelopmental Windows: Implications For Brain Disorders. *Trends in Molecular Medicine, 20*(9), 509–518. https://doi.org/10.1016/j.molmed.2014.05.002

Brazier, Y. (2017, July 28). *How much salt should a person eat?* Medical News Today. https://www.medicalnewstoday.com/articles/146677

Bristol Stool Chart NHS. (2022, December 17). https://bristolstoolchart.info/

Brown, K. (2021, December 10). *How processed foods can affect your health.* Verywell Fit. https://www.verywellfit.com/processed-food-3898404

Bryant, N. (2020, August 15). *The number of calories does muscle burn when compared with fat.* Noah Strength. noahstrength.com/weight-management/the-number-of-calories-does-muscle-burn-when/.

Busch, S. (2018, December 14). *Do humans convert vitamin K1 to vitamin K2?* Week& https://healthyeating.sfgate.com/humans-convert-vitamin-k1-vitamin-k2-11895.html

REFERENCES

Campbell, T. M. & Campbell, T. C. (2016). *What should I eat for my specific condition?* Taking Charge. https://www.takingcharge.csh.umn.edu/what-should-i-eat-my-specific-condition

Carbohydrates and Blood Sugar. (n.d.). https://www.hsph.harvard.edu/nutritionsource/carbohydrates/carbohydrates-and-blood-sugar/

Carrington, D. (2019, June 10). *"Frightening" number of plant extinctions found in global survey.* The Guardian. https://www.theguardian.com/environment/2019/jun/10/frightening-number-of-plant-extinctions-found-in-global-survey

Carter, J. S., Hunter, R. G., Blackston, W. J., Liu, N., Lefkowitz, J. E., Van Der Pol, J. W., Morrow, D. C., Paulsen, A. J., & Rogers, Q. L. (2019). Gut Microbiota Diversity is Associated With Cardiorespiratory Fitness in Post-Primary Treatment Breast Cancer Survivors. *Experimental Physiology, 104*(4), 529–539. https://doi.org/10.1113/ep087404

Cassetty, S. (2019, June 30). *What exactly is a processed meat? And how much is safe to eat?* NBC News. https://www.nbcnews.com/better/lifestyle/what-exactly-processed-meat-how-much-safe-eat-ncna1023401

CDC. (n.d.). Poor nutrition. https://www.cdc.gov/chronicdisease/resources/publications/factsheets/nutrition.htm

Herbs Are the Friend of the Physician and the Pride of Cooks. (n.d.). quotefancy.com/quote/1710220/Charlemagne-Herbs-are-the-friend-of-the-physician-and-the-pride-of-cooks.

Choline. (2022, June 2). https://ods.od.nih.gov/factsheets/Choline-HealthProfessional/

Classification of Vegetables: 9 Categories. (2016, July 22). Your Article Library. https://www.yourarticlelibrary.com/vegetables/classification-of-vegetables-9-categories/86419

Clear, J. (2018). *Atomic habits: an easy & proven way to build good habits & break bad ones.* Avery.

Coast Packing Company. (2016, June 29). *Consumers read food labels, but don't always understand or trust them, new coast packing/ipsos survey reveals.* Cision PR Newswire. https://www.prnewswire.com/news-releases/consumers-read-food-labels-but-dont-always-understand-or-trust-them-new-coast-packingipsos-survey-reveals-300291564.html

Cognitive behavioural therapy can provide better long-term relief for IBS symptoms than current standard treatment. (2019, April 11). University of Southampton. https://www.southampton.ac.uk/news/2019/04/ibs-cbt-treatment.page

Collyer-Smith, J. (2015, April 26). *Western diet impacts on gut health.* Probiotics Learning Lab. https://www.optibacprobiotics.com/learning-lab/in-depth/general-health/western-diet-linked-less-diverse-gut-bacteria

REFERENCES

Conklin, A. Q., Crosswell, D. A., Saron, D. C., & Epel, S. E. (2019). Meditation, Stress Processes, and Telomere Biology. *Current Opinion in Psychology, 28,* 92–101. https://doi.org/10.1016/j.copsyc.2018.11.009

Coolidge, L. F. & Wynn, T. (2013, November 22). *The truth about the caveman diet.* Psychology Today. https://www.psychologytoday.com/us/blog/how-think-neandertal/201311/the-truth-about-the-caveman-diet

Creveling, M. (2023, January 6). *Does exercising boost your immune system?* Health. https://www.health.com/fitness/does-exercise-boost-immunity

Crouch, M. (2023, April 13). *How two minutes of exercise can help you live longer.* AARP. https://www.aarp.org/health/healthy-living/info-2021/exercise-and-longevity.html

Curry, A. N. & Kasser, T. (2011). *Can Coloring Mandalas Reduce Anxiety?* Art Therapy, 22(2), 81–85. https://doi.org/10.1080/07421656.2005.10129441

Daniells, S. (2009, May 26). *Multivitamins linked to younger "biological age": Study.* Nutraingredients. https://www.nutraingredients-usa.com/Article/2009/05/27/Multivitamins-linked-to-younger-biological-age-Study

David, M. (1994). *Nourishing wisdom: a mind-body approach to nutrition and well-being.* Harmony.

Davis, A. (1988). *Let's eat right to keep fit.* Signet Press.

De Francesco, V., Zullo, A., Manta, R., Luigi, G., Giulia, F., Ilaria, M, S., & Dino, V. (2021). Helicobacter Pylori Eradication Following First-Line Treatment Failure in Europe: What, How and When Chose Among Different Standard Regimens? A Systematic Review. *European Journal of Gastroenterology & Hepatology, 33*(1S), e66–e70. https://doi.org/10.1097/MEG.0000000000002100

Dellwo, A. (2022, November 23). *Long-term effects of antidepressants.* Verywell Mind. https://www.verywellmind.com/long-term-effects-of-antidepressants-4158064

Diet and mental health. (2022, January 25). https://www.mentalhealth.org.uk/explore-mental-health/a-z-topics/diet-and-mental-health

Dobrić, M. (2020, January 4). *31 alarming high blood pressure statistics for 2023.* Health Careers. https://healthcareers.co/high-blood-pressure-statistics/#:~:text=It%E2%80%99s%20estimated%20that%20more%20than%20972%20million%20people

DoctorNDTV. (2019, January 29). *An egg a day can keep heart disease away; other health benefits of eggs.* NDTV. https://www.ndtv.com/health/an-egg-a-day-can-keep-heart-disease-away-heres-how-other-health-benefits-of-eggs-1984430

Dorfner, M. (2016, December 13). *Helpful ways you can reduce your sodium intake.* Mayo Clinic News Network. https://newsnetwork.mayoclinic.org/discussion/helpful-ways-you-can-reduce-your-sodium-intake/

REFERENCES

Ducharme, J. (2019, May 15). *Are onions and garlic healthy? Here's what experts say.* Time. https://time.com/5566916/are-garlic-and-onions-healthy/

Duhigg, C. (2014). *The power of habit: why we do what we do and how to change.* Random House Trade Paperbacks.

Eatingwell Editors. (2023, March 16). *The Dirty Dozen: 12 Foods You Should Buy Organic.* EatingWell. www.eatingwell.com/article/15806/the-dirty-dozen-12-foods-you-should-buy-organic/.

EcoWatch. (2016, May 6). *5 ways eating processed foods messes with your body.* https://www.ecowatch.com/5-ways-eating-processed-foods-messes-with-your-body-1891128657.html

8 lifestyle habits destroying your gut health. (2021, October 11). https://gutperformance.com.au/8-lifestyle-habits-destroying-your-gut-health/

11 foods that lower cholesterol. (2021, August 13). https://www.health.harvard.edu/heart-health/11-foods-that-lower-cholesterol

11 types of cheese that contain probiotics. (2022, August 4). Fermenters Kitchen. https://fermenterskitchen.com/11-types-of-cheese-that-contain-probiotics/

Elston, D. M. (2019). Confirmation Bias in Medical Decision-Making. *Journal of the American Academy of Dermatology, 82*(3), 572. https://doi.org/10.1016/j.jaad.2019.06.1286

Erickson, J. M. (2021, April 5). *Turmeric and Osteoarthritis.* Handcare. https://www.assh.org/handcare/blog/turmeric-and-osteoarthritis

Eske, J. (2023, February 10). *Health benefits of coconut milk.* Medical News Today. https://www.medicalnewstoday.com/articles/323743

EU Versus US: A Closer Look at Food Standards. (2018, February 20). http://www.germinalorganic.com/2018/02/eu-versus-us-a-closer-look-at-food-standards/

Faecal therapy back in vogue to treat superbugs. (2013, February 11). https://www.abc.net.au/radionational/programs/ockhamsrazor/poo-therapy/4512736

Fairtrade is the most recognized ethical label in the world. (n.d.). https://www.fairtradeamerica.org/

Falcon, A. (2006, January 11). *Aristotle on causality.* Standford Encyclopedia of Philosophy. https://plato.stanford.edu/entries/aristotle-causality/

Fanelli, M. S., Jonnalagadda, S. S., Pisegna, L. J., Kelly, J. O., Krok-Schoen, L. J., & Taylor, A. C. (2020). Poorer Diet Quality Observed Among US Adults With a Greater Number of Clinical Chronic Disease Risk Factors. *Journal of Primary Care & Community Health, 11.* https://doi.org/10.1177/2150132720945898

Farhud, D. D. (2015). Impact of Lifestyle on Health. *Iranian Journal of Public Health, 44*(11), 1442–1444. https://www.ncbi.nlm.nih.gov/pmc/articles/PMC4703222/

REFERENCES

Fats and Cholesterol. (n.d.). https://www.hsph.harvard.edu/nutritionsource/what-should-you-eat/fats-and-cholesterol/

Fats and oils. (n.d.). https://www.heartuk.org.uk/low-cholesterol-foods/fats-and-oils

Fields, H. (n.d.). *The gut: where bacteria and immune system meet.* John Hopkins Medicine. https://www.hopkinsmedicine.org/research/advancements-in-research/fundamentals/in-depth/the-gut-where-bacteria-and-immune-system-meet

Five Factors that Affect the Immune System. (2021, January 4). https://www.kemin.com/na/en-us/blog/human-nutrition/five-factors-that-affect-immune-system

Fletcher, J. (2020, January 17). *What are fat-soluble vitamins?* Medical News Today. https://www.medicalnewstoday.com/articles/320310#vitamin-e

Food as Preventative Medicine. (n.d.). https://foodforhealth.techno-science.ca/health-and-nutrition/food-as-preventative-medicine/

Food is Medicine Coalition. (n.d.). https://www.fimcoalition.org/

Food processing and nutrition. (n.d.) https://www.betterhealth.vic.gov.au/health/healthyliving/food-processing-and-nutrition

Food sources of vitamin D. (n.d.). https://www.dietaryguide
    lines.gov/resources/2020-2025-dietary-guidelines-online-
    materials/food-sources-select-nutrients/food-sources#:~:text
    =Food%20Sources%20of%20Vitamin%20D%20%20

Forest Bathing. (2022, May 13). https://www.psychology
    today.com/ca/basics/forest-bathing

Fuhrman, J. (2011). *Super immunity: The essential nutrition guide for boosting your body's defenses to live longer, stronger, and disease free.* HarperOne.

Giampapa, V. (2019, October 17). *The complete guide to vegan protein and amino acids.* Healthycell. https://www.healthycell.com/blogs/articles/guide-to-vegan-protein-and-amino-acids

Gibbons, A. (n.d.). *Could eating like our ancestors make us healthier?* National Geographic. https://www.national geographic.com/foodfeatures/evolution-of-diet/

Gluten: a benefit or harm to the body? (n.d.). https://www.hsph.harvard.edu/nutritionsource/gluten/

Goodreads. (n.d.). *Jack Lalanne > Quotes > Quotable Quote.* https://www.goodreads.com/quotes/206315-exercise-is-king-nutrition-is-queen-put-them-together-and

Goodwin, J. (2019, June 17). *The time to relax is when you don't have time for it.* Westgate Resorts. https://www.westgat eresorts.com/blog/time-to-relax-is-when-you-dont-have-time-for-it/#:~:text=%2D%20Jim%20Goodwin

REFERENCES

Gøtzsche, P. C., Smith, R., & Drummond Rennie. (2013). *Deadly medicines and organised crime: how big pharma has corrupted healthcare.* CRC Press.

Guglielmi, G. (2019, December 6). *How modern life affects the microbiota.* Microbiome Post. https://microbiomepost.com/how-modern-life-affects-the-microbiota/

Guthealthimprovment.com. "19 Gut Health Quotes & Sayings 2023 - Gut Health Improvement | Improve Your Gut Health Naturally." *Guthealthimprovement.com*, 29 Sept. 2022, guthealthimprovement.com/gut-health-quotes/. Accessed 17 May 2023.

Ha, E. (2020, April 20). *Food Marketing.* UConn Rudd Center for Food Policy & Health. https://uconnruddcenter.org/research/food-marketing/

Haghighi, S. A. (2021, April 21). *What is an excessive amount of dietary salt?* Medical News Today. https://www.medicalnewstoday.com/articles/too-much-salt#long-term-complications

Hailey, L. (2021a, June 19). *Why are modern foods less nutritious?* Medium. https://loganhailey.medium.com/why-are-modern-foods-less-nutritious-13052839fd09

Hailey, L. (2021b, June 24). *GMOs, demystified in plain language.* Medium. https://medium.com/age-of-awareness/gmos-demystified-in-plain-language-c446d7eed48b

Harrison, D. (2023, January 12). *11 fruits and vegetables high in vitamin K*. Healthy Food Tribe. https://www.healthyfoodtribe.com/fruits-and-vegetables-high-in-vitamin-k/

Hartley, R. & O'Brien, R. (1973). *Sweet Tranvestite*.

Harvard Health. (2018, December 4). *Vitamins and Minerals*. Helpguide.org. https://www.helpguide.org/harvard/vitamins-and-minerals.htm/#:~:text=Vitamins%20and%20minerals%20are%20considered%20essential%20nutrients%E2%80%94because%20acting

Harvard Health Publishing. (2019, January 31). *Understanding antioxidants*. https://www.health.harvard.edu/staying-healthy/understanding-antioxidants#:~:text=Antioxidants%20neutralize%20free%20radicals%20by,other%20cells%20in%20the%20body.

HealthAid. (2021, August 27). *Interactions between vitamins & minerals*. https://www.healthaid.co.uk/blogs/news/interactions-between-vitamins-minerals

Healthy eating plate. (n.d.). https://www.hsph.harvard.edu/nutritionsource/healthy-eating-plate/

Herbert, F. (1965). *Dune*. Chilton Books.

Higuera, V. (2017, December 20). *The MIND Diet for Alzheimer's Prevention*. Everyday Health. https://www.everydayhealth.com/diet-and-nutrition/diet/mind-diet-can-this-diet-plan-help-reverse-alzheimers-disease/

REFERENCES

Hippocrates. (2004, April 9). https://en.wikiquote.org/wiki/Hippocrates

Hippocratic Oath - Classic. (n.d.). https://mccolloughscholars.as.ua.edu/hippocratic-oath-classic/

History.com Editors. (2018, January 5). *Hunter-gatherers.* History. https://www.history.com/topics/prehistory/hunter-gatherers

Holmes, A. (2016, April 4). *Gut bacteria: the inside story.* Australian Academy of Science. https://www.science.org.au/curious/people-medicine/gut-bacteria

Hormones in meat. (n.d.). https://food.ec.europa.eu/safety/chemical-safety/hormones-meat_en

How much plastic are you really eating? (n.d.). https://caltonnutrition.com/plastic/

Hyman, M. (2010, July 18). *Why treating your symptoms is a recipe for disaster.* Dr. Hyman. https://drhyman.com/blog/2010/07/18/why-treating-your-symptoms-is-a-recipe-for-disaster/

Irvine, M. H. (2021, March 17). *18 foods high in omega-3s for better brain health.* Livestrong.com. https://www.livestrong.com/article/13732199-foods-high-in-omega-3/

Is full-fat milk good for you? (n.d.). https://www.bhf.org.uk/informationsupport/heart-matters-magazine/nutrition/full-fat-dairy

Jamison, K. (1997). *An unquiet mind: a memoir of moods and madness.* Vintage.

Johnson, J. (2022, August 12). *Our guide to the Mediterranean diet.* Medical News Today. https://www.medicalnewstoday.com/articles/324221#snacks

Joseph, M. (2023, January 18). *30 foods high in vitamin E.* Nutrition Advance. https://www.nutritionadvance.com/foods-high-in-vitamin-e/

Kaff, T. (2020, September 28). *Got mylk? A complete guide to plant-based milks & their benefits.* Amazonia. https://www.amazonia.com/blogs/news/plant-based-milks-benefits

Katch, V. (2017, June 18). *Food as medicine.* Michigan Today. https://michigantoday.umich.edu/2017/06/18/food-as-medicine/

Kaur, M., Agarwal, C., & Agarwal, R. (2009). Anticancer and Cancer Chemopreventive Potential of Grape Seed Extract and Other Grape-Based Products. *The Journal of Nutrition, 139*(9), 1806S–1812S. https://doi.org/10.3945/jn.109.106864

Kerkar, P. (2019, April 16). *What are the harmful effects of fertilizers on human health?* PainAssist. https://www.epainassist.com/articles/what-are-the-harmful-effects-of-fertilizers-on-human-health

Kershner, I. (1980). *Star wars: the empire strikes back.*

REFERENCES

Kirkpatrick, B. (2018, May 15). *Epigenetics, nutrition, and our health: how what we eat could affect tags on our DNA.* What Is Epigenetics? https://www.whatisepigenetics.com/epigenetics-nutrition-health-eat-affect-tags-dna/

Klemow, M. K., Bartlow, A., Crawford, J., Kocher, N., Shah, J., & Ritsick, M. (2011). *Medical attributes of st. john's wort (hypericum perforatum).* Nih.gov; CRC Press/Taylor & Francis. https://www.ncbi.nlm.nih.gov/books/NBK92750/

Kloss, K. (2022, July 12). *19 foods high in antioxidants to eat more often.* Livestrong.com. https://www.livestrong.com/article/13764516-foods-high-in-antioxidants/

Kresser, C. (2017, July 19). *The gut flora-food allergies connection.* Kresser Institute. https://kresserinstitute.com/gut-flora-food-allergies-connection/

Kringold, S. (2022). *Aging gracefully for women over 50: dr. steve's guide to help reverse aging, disease, weight gain and energy lost.* Self-published.

Kringold, S. (2022). *Intermittent fasting for women over 50: dr. steve's guide for rapid weight loss, energy, detoxification, diabetes, and anti-aging (dr. steve's guide).* Self-published.

Kubala, J. & Gunnars, K. (2022, January 6). *16 delicious high protein foods.* Healthline. https://www.healthline.com/nutrition/high-protein-foods

Kuo, B., Bhasin, M., Jacquart, J., Scult, A. M., Slipp, L., Riklin, K. I. E., Lepoutre, V., Comosa, N., Norton, B., Dassatti, A.,

Rosenblum, J., Thurler, H. A., Surjanhata, C. B., Hasheminejad, N. N., Kagan, L., Slawsby, E., Rao, R. S., Macklin, A. E., Fricchione, L. G., Benson, H., Libermann A. T., Korzenik, J., & Denninger, W. J. (2015). Genomic and Clinical Effects Associated with a Relaxation Response Mind-Body Intervention in Patients with Irritable Bowel Syndrome and Inflammatory Bowel Disease. *PLOS ONE, 10*(4), e0123861. https://doi.org/10.1371/journal.pone.0123861

Lehman, S. (2021, September 2). *9 Dietary Trace Minerals and What Foods Are High in Them.* VeryWell Fit. https://www.verywellfit.com/dietary-trace-minerals-and-where-to-find-them-2507747

Lehman, S. (2022, May 28). *What makes junk food so tempting.* Verywell Fit. https://www.verywellfit.com/why-you-eat-junk-food-2507661

Lennon, A. (2021, July 19). *Reading, writing, and playing games delay Alzheimer's by 5 years.* Medical News Today. https://www.medicalnewstoday.com/articles/reading-writing-and-playing-games-delay-alzheimers-by-5-years#Clinical-examinations

Let food be thy medicine –hippocrates? (2018, July 17). https://www.drgoodfood.org/en/news/let-food-be-thy-medicine-hippocrates

Lewin, J. (2023, March 15). *Top 5 benefits of green tea.* BBC Good Food. https://www.bbcgoodfood.com/howto/guide/health-benefits-green-tea

REFERENCES

Light, W. D. (2014, June 27). *New prescription drugs: a major health risk with few offsetting advantages.* Harvard University. https://ethics.harvard.edu/blog/new-prescription-drugs-major-health-risk-few-offsetting-advantages

Lois, P. (2017, December 30). *Percentage of lactose intolerance by ethnicity (and geographic region).* Milk Pro Con. https://www.milkprocon.org/lactose-intolerance-ethnicity/

Lowery, M. (2022, May 21). *How to reduce hunger while fasting?* 2 Meal Day. https://2mealday.com/article/how-to-reduce-hunger-while-fasting/#:~:text=There%20are%20two%20main%20reasons%20for%20this%3A%201

Lumen Learning. (n.d.). The Scientific Process. https://courses.lumenlearning.com/waymaker-psychology/chapter/reading-the-scientific-process-replace-content/

Lucas, G. (1977). *Star wars: episode IV - a new hope.*

Macciochi, J. (2020, June 25). *How to build tiny superhumans.* The Gut Stuff. https://thegutstuff.com/how-to-build-tiny-superhumans/

MacGill, M. (2023, February 15). *What are the gut microbiota and human microbiome?* Medical News Today. https://www.medicalnewstoday.com/articles/307998

Machowsky, J. (2017, May 19). *Should I Take Salt During a Marathon?* NYRR. https://www.nyrr.org/run/photos-and-stories/2019/should-i-take-salt-during-a-marathon

Macia, L., Galy, O., & Nanan, H. K. R. (2021). Editorial: Modern Lifestyle and Health: How Changes in the Environment Impacts Immune Function and Physiology. *Frontiers in Immunology, 12*. https://doi.org/10.3389/fimmu.2021.762166

Malhotra, A. (2018, August 30). *Why modern medicine is a major threat to public health.* The Guardian. https://www.theguardian.com/society/2018/aug/30/modern-medicine-major-threat-public-health

Marcene, B. (2021, October 11). *12 amazing health benefits of fermented foods.* Natural Food Series. https://www.naturalfoodseries.com/12-benefits-fermented-foods/

Martel, J. (2023, May 8). *Hyponatremia: understanding low blood sodium.* Healthline. https://www.healthline.com/health/hyponatremia#complications

May, A. (2022, August 25). *Why is the sky blue?* Space.com. https://www.space.com/why-is-the-sky-blue

Mayo Clinic Staff. (2022, May 4). *Fecal occult blood test.* Mayo Clinic. https://www.mayoclinic.org/tests-procedures/fecal-occult-blood-test/about/pac-20394112

McCulloch, M. (2023, February 23). *30 foods high in sodium and what to eat instead.* Healthline. https://www.healthline.com/nutrition/foods-high-in-sodium

McFarland, T. (2020, September 8). *How are B12 supplements made? Where does B12 come from?* I Am Going Vegan. https://www.iamgoingvegan.com/how-are-b12-supplements-made/

REFERENCES

Mcleod, S. (2023, February 14). *Stress, illness and the immune system*. Simply Psychology. https://www.simplypsychology.org/stress-immune.html

Meek, W. (2020, November 19). *The evolutionary psychology of anxiety*. Verywell Mind. https://www.verywellmind.com/evolution-anxiety-1392983

Melville, K. (2020, September 24). *How does nutrient-depleted soil impact our food, and what can we do to fix it?* Chris Kresser. https://chriskresser.com/depletion-of-soil-and-what-can-be-done/

Merz, B. (2021, February 15). *Micronutrients have major impact on health*. Harvard Health Publishing. https://www.health.harvard.edu/staying-healthy/micronutrients-have-major-impact-on-health

Meyer, P. (2012, November 13). *'Jaw Jaw' is better than 'War War': International Security in Cyberspace*. ICT for Peace Foundation. https://ict4peace.org/activities/jaw-jaw-is-better-than-war-war-international-security-in-cyberspace/#:~:text=%E2%80%9CJaw%20Jaw%20is%20better%20than,conduct%20of%20relations%20between%20states.

Micha, R., Peñalvo, L. J., Cudhea, F., Imamura, F., Rehm, D. C., & Mozaffarian, D. (2017). Association Between Dietary Factors and Mortality From Heart Disease, Stroke, and Type 2 Diabetes in the United States. *JAMA, 317*(9), 912–924. https://doi.org/10.1001/jama.2017.0947

Mind Tools Content Team. (n.d.). https://www.mindtools.com/ avn893g/the-holmes-and-rahe-stress-scale

Mitchell, A. P., Trivedi, N. U., Gennarelli, R. L., Chimonas, S., Tabatabai, S. M., Goldberg, J., Diaz, L. A., & Korenstein, D. (2021). Are Financial Payments From the Pharmaceutical Industry Associated With Physician Prescribing? : A Systematic Review. *Annals of Internal Medicine, 174*(3), 353–361. https://doi.org/10.7326/M20-5665

Mitchell, A., & Korenstein, D. (2020, December 4). *Drug companies' payments and gifts affect physicians' prescribing.* STAT. https://www.statnews.com/2020/12/04/drug-companies-payments-gifts-affect-physician-prescribing/

Moncorgé, J. M. (n.d.). *Hippocratic dietetics.* Oldcook. https://www.oldcook.com/en/medieval-hippocratic_dietetics

Mummert, A., Esche, E., Robinson, J., & Armelagos, G. J. (2011). Stature and robusticity during the agricultural transition: Evidence from the bioarchaeological record. *Economics & Human Biology, 9*(3), 284–301. https://doi.org/10.1016/j.ehb.2011.03.004

National Geographic Society. (2022, July 8). *The Development of Agriculture.* https://education.nationalgeographic.org/resource/development-agriculture/

Ng, Q. X., Venkatanarayanan, N., & Ho, C. Y. (2017). Clinical Use of Hypericum Perforatum (St John's Wort) in Depression: A Meta-Analysis. *Journal of Affective Disorders, 210,* 211–221. 10.1016/j.jad.2016.12.048

REFERENCES

NHS. (n.d.). *Calories in alcohol.* https://www.nhs.uk/live-well/alcohol-advice/calories-in-alcohol/

NIH. (2023, May 11). *Circadian Rhythms.* https://nigms.nih.gov/education/fact-sheets/Pages/Circadian-Rhythms.aspx

Nordqvist, J. (2023, March 1). *Everything you need to know about honey.* Medical News Today. https://www.medicalnewstoday.com/articles/264667#properties

Nutrigenomics. The basics. (2018, November 19). https://www.nutritionsociety.org/blog/nutrigenomics-basics

Omega-3: omega-6 balance. (n.d.). https://www.gbhealthwatch.com/Science-Omega3-Omega6.php

Owens, B. (2013, September 6). *Bacteria from lean mice prevent obesity in peers.* Scientific American. https://www.scientificamerican.com/article/bacteria-from-lean-mice-prevent-obesity-in-peers/

Paleolithic societies. (2017). https://www.khanacademy.org/humanities/world-history/world-history-beginnings/origin-humans-early-societies/a/what-were-paleolithic-societies-like

Pariona, A. (2019, June 7). *What are the world's most important staple foods?* WorldAtlas. https://www.worldatlas.com/articles/most-important-staple-foods-in-the-world.html#:~:text=The%20overwhelming%20majority%20of%20global%20staple%20foods%20are

Park, W. (2021, June 9). *How processed foods became so unhealthy*. BBC. https://www.bbc.com/future/article/20210608-what-were-the-first-processed-foods

Pastoralist and farmer-herder conflicts in the sahel. (1944, January 1). https://climate-diplomacy.org/case-studies/pastoralist-and-farmer-herder-conflicts-sahel

Pavid, K. (2021, February 19). *Aspirin, morphine and chemotherapy: the essential medicines powered by plants*. National History Museum. https://www.nhm.ac.uk/discover/essential-medicines-powered-by-plants.html

Phytochemical. (n.d.). Science Direct. https://www.sciencedirect.com/topics/agricultural-and-biological-sciences/phytochemical

Poets.org. (2007, December 19). *Childe Harold's Pilgrimage [There is a pleasure in the pathless woods] by George Gordon Byron*. https://poets.org/poem/childe-harolds-pilgrimage-there-pleasure-pathless-woods

Pratt, E. (2022, November 5). *A guide to gluten-free grains*. Verywell Health. https://www.verywellhealth.com/a-guide-to-gluten-free-grains-5211338

Premier Wellness Centers. (2020, November 19). *How our modern world is stressing our immune system*. https://premierwellnesscenters.com/wellness/how-our-modern-world-is-stressing-our-immune-system/

REFERENCES

Randall, B. (2022, December 5). *The science behind cold water plunges*. Discover Magazine. https://www.discovermagazine.com/health/the-science-behind-cold-water-plunges

Rasmussen, H. E., & Hamaker, B. R. (2017). Prebiotics and Inflammatory Bowel Disease. *Gastroenterology Clinics of North America, 46*(4), 783–795. https://doi.org/10.1016/j.gtc.2017.08.004

Rayner, S. (2018, June 28). *Sick, fat and unhealthy: where did it all go wrong?* The Sustainable Training Method. https://www.thesustainabletrainingmethod.com/tstm-blog/2018/6/26/sick-fat-and-unhealthy-where-did-is-all-go-wrong

Redelmeier, D. A., & Shafir, E. (1995). Medical decision making in situations that offer multiple alternatives. *JAMA, 273*(4), 302–305. https://pubmed.ncbi.nlm.nih.gov/7815657/

Retno, P. (2017, May 18). *24 best health benefits of sea salt (#1 top mineral source)*. DrHealthBenefits.com. https://drhealthbenefits.com/food-bevarages/flavourings/health-benefits-of-sea-salt

Robertson, M. D., Bickerton, A. S., Dennis, A. L., Vidal, H., & Frayn, K. N. (2005). Insulin-sensitizing effects of dietary resistant starch and effects on skeletal muscle and adipose tissue metabolism. *The American Journal of Clinical Nutrition, 82*(3), 559–567. https://doi.org/10.1093/ajcn.82.3.559

Robertson, S. (2019, December 4). *Can you treat a food allergy by altering the gut microbiome?* News Medical Life Sciences. https://www.news-medical.net/health/Can-you-Treat-a-Food-Allergy-by-Altering-the-Gut-Microbiome.aspx

Ruggeri, C. (2022, March 23). *Top 17 foods high in zinc (& their health benefits)*. Dr. Axe. https://draxe.com/nutrition/foods-high-in-zinc/

Russel, J. (2023, April 20). *Visual cliff experiment (Gibson and Walk, 1960)*. Simply Psychology. https://www.simplypsychology.org/visual-cliff-experiment.html

Ruth, Angela. *Dickens Quote - Debt Results in Misery.* (2022, June 13). *Due*. due.com/dickens-quote-debt-results-in-misery/#:~:text=Charles%20Dickens%20often%20made%20references%20of%20the%20consequences.

Ryan, A. (2023, April 12). *Are air fryers healthy?* Medical News Today. https://www.medicalnewstoday.com/articles/324849#summary

Sager, Jessica. (2021, June 5). *60 doctor who quotes from all 13 doctors to make you feel better about your place in the universe*. Parade. parade.com/1218758/jessicasager/doctor-who-quotes/

Salomon, H. S. (2021, March 1). *Food as medicine: what it means and how to reap the benefits*. Everyday Health. https://www.everydayhealth.com/diet-nutrition/food-as-medicine-what-it-means-and-how-to-reap-the-benefits/

Seow, S. (2023, February 13). *These 12 healthy foods are exceptionally high in vitamin B*. Real Simple. https://www.realsimple.com/health/nutrition-diet/vitamin-b-foods

REFERENCES

Servick, K. (2019, May 16). *"Ultraprocessed" foods may make you eat more, clinical trial suggests.* Science. https://www.science.org/content/article/ultraprocessed-foods-may-make-you-eat-more-clinical-trial-suggests

7 health benefits of turmeric. (2021, November 10). https://health.clevelandclinic.org/turmeric-health-benefits/

Shapiro, S. C. (2018, November 19). *Turmeric: the evidence for therapeutic use for arthritis.* The Rheumatologist. https://www.the-rheumatologist.org/article/turmeric-the-evidence-for-therapeutic-use-for-arthritis/

Sharma, A., Sabharwal, P., & Dada, R. (2021, January 1). *Chapter 1 - Herbal medicine—An introduction to its history.* ScienceDirect; Academic Press. https://www.sciencedirect.com/science/article/abs/pii/B9780128155653000011

Shaw, G. (2011, June 27). *Is your diet aging you?* WebMD. https://www.webmd.com/diet/features/is-your-diet-aging-you

Shelley, M. (1818). *Frankenstein.* Beverly, Ma Rockport Publishers.

Should I take a daily multivitamin? (2021, July). https://www.hsph.harvard.edu/nutritionsource/multivitamin/

Should you eat a rainbow of fruits and vegetables? (2017, July 20). https://www.bhf.org.uk/informationsupport/heart-matters-magazine/nutrition/5-a-day/colourful-foods

Simran. (2023, April 25). *Sleep psychologists: improving your sleep habits for a healthy life.* Mantra Care. https://mantracare.org/therapy/psychologist/sleep-psychologists/

16 best antiviral herbs and supplements to boost your immune system and keep you healthy. (2022, November 10). https://www.medicinenet.com/16_best_antiviral_herbs_supplements_boost_immune/article.htm

Small beer. (2001, November 4). https://en.wikipedia.org/wiki/Small_beer

Smith, R. P., Easson, C., Lyle, S. M., Kapoor, R., Donnelly, C. P., Davidson, E. J., Parikh, E., Lopez, J. V., & Tartar, J. L. (2019). Gut microbiome diversity is associated with sleep physiology in humans. *PLOS ONE, 14*(10). https://doi.org/10.1371/journal.pone.0222394

Sowndhararajan, K., & Kim, S. (2016). Influence of Fragrances on Human Psychophysiological Activity: With Special Reference to Human Electroencephalographic Response. *Scientia Pharmaceutica, 84*(4), 724–751. https://doi.org/10.3390/scipharm84040724

Spector, T. (2020). *Spoon-fed: why almost everything we've been told about food is wrong.* Jonathan Cape.

Spritzler, F. (2023, April 12). *Ghee: healthier than regular butter?* Healthline. https://www.healthline.com/nutrition/ghee#potential-downsides

Staab, J. (2021, March 9). *What makes superfood so super?* UC Davis. https://www.ucdavis.edu/food/what-makes-superfood-so-super

REFERENCES

Staff. New (2018, November 13). *Physical activity guidelines for americans.* Harvard T.H. Chan. https://www.hsph.harvard.edu/nutritionsource/2018/11/13/new-physical-activity-guidelines-for-americans/

Stewart, L. (2019, September 11). *Top 5 gut bacteria with unusual health benefits.* Atlas Biomed Blog. https://atlasbiomed.com/blog/top-5-gut-bacteria-with-unusual-health-benefits/

Strickler, L. (2021, July 20). *4 drug companies agree to pay $26 billion to resolve opioid lawsuits.* NBC News. https://www.nbcnews.com/news/us-news/4-companies-near-26-billion-settlement-resolve-opioid-lawsuits-n1274520

Sturluson, T. (2014, January 30). *History of herbal medicine.* The Herbal Resource. https://www.herbal-supplement-resource.com/history-of-herbal-medicine/

Suglia, E. (2018, December 10). *Vanishing Nutrients.* Scientific American. https://blogs.scientificamerican.com/observations/vanishing-nutrients/

Sunlight offers surprise benefit: It energizes infection fighting T cells. (2016, December 20). Science Daily. https://www.sciencedaily.com/releases/2016/12/161220094633.htm

Super User. (2005, February 1). *A focus on natural COX-2 inhibitors.* Sabinsa. https://sabinsa.com/newsletters-december-2004-january-2005/589-a-focus-on-natural-cox-2-inhibitors

Swanson, R. (2006, November 15). *Dark chocolate lowers blood clot risk*. Medical News Today. https://www.medicalnewstoday.com/articles/56788#1

NIH (2018). *Vitamins and minerals*. https://www.nccih.nih.gov/health/vitamins-and-minerals#:~:text=A%20number%20of%20minerals%20are,fluoride%2C%20manganese%2C%20and%20selenium.

The dawn of agriculture. (n.d.). https://www.khanacademy.org/humanities/world-history/world-history-beginnings/birth-agriculture-neolithic-revolution/a/where-did-agriculture-come-from

The Doctor of the Future. (2017, June 5). https://evidenceinmotion.com/the-doctor-of-the-future/

The environmental and health impacts of growth hormones in cattle rearing. (2013, December 11). https://www.organic-center.org/research/environmental-and-health-impacts-growth-hormones-cattle-rearing

The Isthmus. *The power of the gut, outside of the gut*. (2016, May 13). Medium.https://medium.com/the-isthmus/the-power-of-the-gut-outside-of-the-gut-92e071e308f3#:~:text=%E2%80%9CThe%20gut%20is%20not%20like,not%20stay%20in%20the%20gut.%E2%80%9D&text=There%20was%20once%20a%20time,disorders%2C%20like%20bloating%20and%20constipation.

The Time to Relax Is When You Don't Have Time for It – Quote Investigator®. *Quoteinvestigator.com*, 13 Jan. 2022, quoteinvestigator.com/2022/01/13/relax-time/. Accessed 17 May 2023.

REFERENCES

The Top Boron Rich Foods Sources. (n.d.). https://www.algae cal.com/algaecal-ingredients/boron/boron-sources/#:~:text=%20%20%20%20Food%20%20%20

Theodosius Dobzhansky Quotes. (n.d.). https://www.goodreads.com/author/quotes/8073211.Theodosius_Dobzhansky

Thomée, S., Härenstam, A., & Hagberg, M. (2011). Mobile phone use and stress, sleep disturbances, and symptoms of depression among young adults - a prospective cohort study. *BMC Public Health, 11*(1). https://doi.org/10.1186/1471-2458-11-66

Tikkanen, R. & Abrams, M. K. (2020, January 30). *U.S. health care from a global perspective, 2019: higher spending, worse outcomes?* The Commonwealth Fund. https://www.commonwealthfund.org/publications/issue-briefs/2020/jan/us-health-care-global-perspective-2019

Tom of AskaNaturalist.com. (2010, November 17). *Which cells are never replaced?* AskaNaturalist.com. https://askanaturalist.com/which-cells-are-never-replaced/

Totelin, L. (2015). When foods become remedies in ancient Greece: The curious case of garlic and other substances. *Journal of Ethnopharmacology, 167*, 30–37. https://doi.org/10.1016/j.jep.2014.08.018

Tucker, A. & Todd, C. L. (2022, July 30). *47 healthy snack ideas that'll get you out of your rut.* SELF. https://www.self.com/gallery/14-healthy-snacks-that-you-can-and-should-keep-at-your-desk

Tweed, V. (2021, September 21). *The 100-year history of vitamins.* Better Nutrition. https://www.betternutrition.com/supplements/vitamins/history-of-vitamins/

22 calcium-rich foods to try right now. (2022, May 2). https://health.clevelandclinic.org/calcium-rich-foods/

U.S. Department of Health and Human Services. (2018). *Physical Activity Guidelines for Americans.* https://health.gov/sites/default/files/2019-09/Physical_Activity_Guidelines_2nd_edition.pdf

USDA says ORAC tests useless, removes database for selected foods. (2012, June 12). Natural Products Insider. https://www.naturalproductsinsider.com/claims/usda-says-orac-tests-useless-removes-database-selected-foods

USDA. (2020). *Dietary Guidelines for Americans.* https://www.dietaryguidelines.gov/sites/default/files/2020-12/Dietary_Guidelines_for_Americans_2020-2025.pdf

Van De Walle, G. (2018, December 5). *How much sodium should you have per day?* Healthline. https://www.healthline.com/nutrition/sodium-per-day#recommendations

Van Oord, G. (2019, July 17). *The gut-brain axis explained in plain english.* Diet vs Disease. https://www.dietvsdisease.org/gut-brain-axis/

Vedantu. (2023, May 8). *Ptyalin.* https://www.vedantu.com/biology/ptyalin

Vegetables and Fruits. (n.d.). https://www.hsph.harvard.edu/nutritionsource/what-should-you-eat/vegetables-and-fruits/

REFERENCES

Villines, Z. (2021, November 17). *Is ADHD overdiagnosed and overtreated?* Medical News Today. https://www.medicalnewstoday.com/articles/is-adhd-overdiagnosed-and-overtreated

Vitamins and minerals. (n.d.). https://www.hsph.harvard.edu/nutritionsource/vitamins/

Wallace, R. (2007). *Maxey-rosenau-last public health and preventive medicine* (15th Edition). Mcgraw-Hill Medical.

Want to know how long you will live? Count your teeth! (2015, April 30). https://www.dentalhealth.org/News/want-to-know-how-long-you-will-live-count-your-teeth

Weaver, J. (2021, July 12). *A fermented-food diet increases microbiome diversity and lowers inflammation, study finds.* Stanford Medicine. https://med.stanford.edu/news/all-news/2021/07/fermented-food-diet-increases-microbiome-diversity-lowers-inflammation

Wedro, B. (2016, November 10). *Blood Doping.* MedicineNet. https://www.medicinenet.com/blood_doping/views.htm

Weldzius, A. (2022, April 13). *6 ways how processed food effect your body.* Lit Medical. https://litmedical.net/6-ways-how-processed-food-effect-your-body/

What happens to your body when you don't get enough sleep (and how much you really need a night). (2022, March 25). https://health.clevelandclinic.org/happens-body-dont-get-enough-sleep/

Whole-grains. (n.d.). https://www.hsph.harvard.edu/nutritionsource/what-should-you-eat/whole-grains/

Why good nutrition is important. (n.d.). https://www.cspinet.org/eating-healthy/why-good-nutrition-important

Why real food is no longer enough. (2016, June 6). https://caltonnutrition.com/real-food-is-simply-not-enough/

William Shakespeare Quote. (n.d.). libquotes.com/william-shakespeare/quote/lbi6j1y. Accessed 17 May 2023.

Wilson, B. (2019, March 16). *Good enough to eat? The toxic truth about modern food.* The Guardian. https://www.theguardian.com/books/2019/mar/16/snack-attacks-the-toxic-truth-about-the-way-we-eat

Wolfe, V. (1929). *A room of one's own.* Hogarth Press.

Wunsch, N. (2020, November 25). *Estimated value of probiotics market worldwide from 2018 to 2023.* Statista. https://www.statista.com/statistics/821259/global-probioticsl-market-value/

Yogi, P. (2016, March 21). *Loftus and Palmer (1974) - Eyewitness Testimony.* Psych Yogi. http://psychyogi.org/loftus-and-palmer-1974-eyewitness-testimony/

Younkin, L. (2020, April 15). *Hormone-balancing foods: how your diet can help keep your hormones functioning well.* Eating Well. https://www.eatingwell.com/article/7805452/hormone-balancing-foods-how-diet-can-help/